STROKE REHABILITATION

STROKE REHABILITATION

A Guide to the Rehabilitation of an Adult Patient Following a Stroke

By

HARRY T. ZANKEL, M.D.

Former Consultant in Physical Medicine and Rehabilitation
Veterans Administration Hospital
Columbia, South Carolina
Former Chief, Physical Medicine and Reconditioning
U. S. Army Hospitals
Former Chief, Physical Medicine and Rehabilitation
Veterans Administration Hospitals
Cleveland, Ohio; Durham, North Carolina;
and Columbia, South Carolina

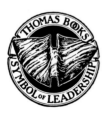

CHARLES C THOMAS • PUBLISHER
Springfield • *Illinois* • *U.S.A.*

Published and Distributed Througout the World by
CHARLES C THOMAS • PUBLISHER
BANNERSTONE HOUSE
301-327 East Lawrence Avenue, Springfield, Illinois, U.S.A.

NATCHEZ PLANTATION HOUSE
735 North Atlantic Boulevard, Fort Lauderdale, Florida, U.S.A.

With THOMAS BOOKS *careful attention is given to all details of*
manufacturing and design. It is the Publisher's desire to present books
that are satisfactory as to their physical qualities and artistic possibilities
and appropriate for their particular use. THOMAS BOOKS *will be true*
to those laws of quality that assure a good name and good will.

Printed in the United States of America
PP-22

To My Daughters
Isralea Efroymson and Esther Yanof

PREFACE

One of my duties as Chief, Physical Medicine and Rehabilitation of the Veterans Administration Hospital, Columbia, South Carolina, was to inspect nursing homes for approval by the Veterans Administration to determine if they were suitable for our veterans who needed such placement. It was discouraging to see so many inmates obviously suffering from the residuals of a stroke, lying in bed or sitting in a wheelchair, apparently given up as hopeless nursing care problems. It was obvious to me that many of them had not received, and were still not receiving, the attention which they deserved. Hence, when Mr. Payne Thomas invited me to write a monograph on the rehabilitation of a patient following a stroke, I readily agreed. Perhaps too readily, for, as I began to review the literature, I was overwhelmed by its enormity. Yet, in spite of the innumerable articles and many books written on "stroke," there so far has not been published one book or monograph on the salient features of stroke rehabilitation. This is one reason for the present volume.

The other reason is that for the past forty years or so, at first in private practice, then during the Second World War in the Army, and for the past twenty-five years in the Veterans Administration, I have been studying, caring for, and doing research on stroke patients, and teaching professional personnel and patients. While most of the teaching and treatment have been in line with the general professional approaches, I have developed some ideas of my own and should like to share them with my readers. The stroke 4-dys syndrome, the S.A.E. routine, the pallesthesia studies in stroke patients are examples of what I have incorporated in this book. In a word, what I have attempted now is a practical guide to the rehabilitation of a patient following a stroke. I hope that my ideas and the general arrangement will be of benefit to the students and members of the medical and allied professions, as well as to the intelligent public.

HARRY T. ZANKEL

vii

INTRODUCTION

My definition of rehabilitation is the following: Rehabilitation is a program of treatment and activity, the purpose of which is to restore to a patient in the shortest feasible time, the maximum physical, mental, social, and if possible, vocational health, with a view to rendering him most useful to himself and society. How does this apply to stroke rehabilitation?

When a young healthy carpenter has an accident resulting in a leg amputation, he is given stump conditioning and preprosthetic training; he is fitted with an artificial limb and trained in its use. He goes back to work, either as a carpenter or into some other suitable trade. He is rehabilitated in the true sense of the word. A young mechanic of thirty or so is operated on for a berry aneurism, develops a stroke, makes a good recovery, except for residual weakness in the left upper extremity, and goes back to his mechanic's work. He too may be said to be rehabilitated. But take an older man or woman with cerebrovascular disease who develops a right hemiplegia and dysphasia. After a prolonged program of treatment and training, he or she is able to walk with a cane, to express himself or herself, and to take care of his or her daily needs. Can we say that he or she is rehabilitated? Not as long as the cerebrovascular disease has not been ameliorated. The best we can say is that we have assisted the patient in attaining maximum recovery in view of his disability, always remembering that in the offing lurks another stroke. With this understanding, we shall proceed with development of our monograph, always keeping in mind that when we say the patient is rehabilitated, we mean with regards to the particular incident for which he was treated.

The object of this monograph, therefore, is to indicate those measures that will provide maximum recovery to a patient following a stroke, realizing all the time that, in doing so, we (that is, the rehabilitation team) have brought the patient to his maximum usefulness to himself and society in view of his current episode.

In the chapters to follow we shall analyze the general considerations pertinent to the subject, including some principles, as well as early treatment. We shall devote a whole section to the various manifestations of what I like to call the *stroke 4-dys syndrome:* dyskinesia, dysesthesia, dysphasia, and dysmentia. Then we shall review the various barriers or hindrances that make it difficult to obtain a good rehabilitation result. This will be followed by an outline of the self-care activities and self-help devices applicable particularly to a one-handed individual. The *stroke rehabilitation team* will be discussed as to makeup and function. The book will conclude with a brief review of present status and future prospects in stroke rehabilitation. For those interested in teaching and demonstrating, I have inserted in the Appendix a dramatization of a patient following a stroke. I call it a *phystheatric* demonstration. It is printed exactly as produced over Station WUNC-TV, Chapel Hill, North Carolina.

I have aimed primarily for a practical manual on stroke rehabilitation. Although some salient features of diagnosis and treatment may be mentioned in passing, the primary consideration will be given to rehabilitation rather than to definitive diagnosis and treatment.

The reader will also note that I have avoided the use of the words "involved" and "uninvolved," and "normal" and "abnormal" when referring to the extremities of the stroke patient. I prefer to use the terms "paretic" or "paralytic" upper or lower extremity versus the "nonparetic" upper or lower extremity, since in the usual stroke there is some involvement in all extremities.

I have also tried to make each part more or less complete in itself so that the reader does not have constantly to refer back and forth to some of the salient items discussed.

I shall conclude this introduction by giving my definition of a stroke. A *stroke* is a focal brain lesion in a patient who has been suffering from cerebrovascular disease. The disease may be intracranial as, for example, cerebral arteriosclerosis, or extracranial, such as is seen in vertebral or carotid artery constriction. In other words, a stroke is an incident in cerebrovascular disease or, as it is usually called, a cerebrovascular accident, or a C.V.A.   H.T.Z.

ACKNOWLEDGMENTS

A book, certainly a medical book, is not composed entirely out of the pure imagination of the author. A play perhaps is, but a scientific manual? Hardly. This is true of the present volume. It is not only fair, but just, that acknowledgment be made of the more important ingredients blended into the present monograph. Probably the first one for me to thank is Mr. Payne Thomas, but for whose invitation this book would never have been written. It was he who suggested the book as well as the title. Next, I should like to thank the innumerable writers of books and articles who together and separately helped to shape this volume. In many cases I have tried to indicate them by reference which the reader will find at the end of the book. Special mention in this respect should be made of the American Heart Association and the American Rehabilitation Foundation who have done so much in the dissemination of information on stroke and its management. Mr. Verne Atkinson, Director of Medical Illustrations of the Columbia Veterans Administration Hospital, who did such a fine job with the illustrations, deserves commendation. Thanks should also be given to the many patients and personnel whose photos make up the bulk of the illustrations. Finally, a word of special appreciation to the members of the rehabilitation team whom I have taught and who, in turn, have taught me the practical procedures in the rehabilitation of a patient following a stroke.

H.T.Z.

CONTENTS

PART III
BARRIERS TO STROKE REHABILITATION

PART IV
ACTIVITIES OF DAILY LIVING

PART V
THE STROKE REHABILITATION TEAM

STROKE REHABILITATION

PART I
GENERAL CONSIDERATIONS

Chapter 1

EPIDEMIOLOGY

I n 1965, over 200,000 people in the United States died of a stroke, as compared with 1,825,000 who died from all causes.[1] This is a stroke mortality rate of over 11 percent. In fact, stroke is the third largest cause of death, next only to heart disease and cancer. The number of stroke deaths per 100,000 population has remained fairly constant in recent years. The ratio per 100,000 of all deaths is 941.6 and of stroke deaths is 104.9. Eighty percent of stroke deaths, i.e. 160,000 per year, occur in people over 65 and 20 percent, i.e. 40,000 per year, in people under 65. The incidence of stroke and its consequences may be expected to increase with the increase of longevity.

Two thousand years ago, the average length of life was 25 years. Today, it is 67 for males and 72.4 for females.

The largest single number of deaths, i.e. over 73,000, occurred in the 75-84 age group. As regards sex, stroke, unlike heart disease or cancer, claims more female than male victims in the United States, 107,000 versus 94,000. Nonwhite females have the highest death rate from strokes, but the death rate for white females is lower than that for white males.

According to the President's Commission on Heart Disease, Cancer, and Stroke,[2] there is a definite geographical pattern for stroke death rates, the highest death rates occurring in the southeastern states and the lowest in the southwestern and mountain regions.

Eight of ten stroke victims survive the acute phase. Most of these require assistance with their daily needs because they have not been exposed to a good rehabilitation program. About 300,000, whose primary diagnosis is stroke, are discharged annually from the nation's short-term hospitals. In nursing homes, 16 percent of all patients are suffering from stroke residuals.

The cost is staggering. In 1962, direct expenditure for services and supplies for stroke management amounted to 440 million dollars. The total economic cost was given as 1.1 billion dollars. With present rise in medical and hospital costs and the general rise in cost of living, the figures for the seventies will be much greater.

If we go back to the fifties, the stroke death rate per 100,000 population in the United States[3] was 108.5 for white males and females, the figure for males being 104.8 and for females, 112. For nonwhites, the rate for both sexes was 123.4, 121.8 for males and 124.8 for females. According to Goldberg and Curland,[4] in the fifties the United States *nonwhite* population, next to Japan, led all other countries in mortality statistics for vascular lesions of the nervous system, i.e. 164.6 per 100,000 as compared with a *white* mortality in the U.S. of 94.8. Combining the whites and nonwhites, the mortality was 101.4 per 100,000. There was marked variation in mortality rates in other countries, for example, 16.8 per 100,000 in the Philippines to 208.6 per 100,000 in Japan; and 116.2 in England and Wales; 149.9 in West Germany; 98.5 in France; and only 48.3 in its neighbor, Belgium. However, it should be noted that these marked differences may in part be due to the manner of coding.

For example, Katsuki *et al.*,[5] studying a group of 1,841 patients over forty years of age, lost 56 in eighteen months. There were 30.4 percent autopsies. Cerebrovascular deaths exceeded those due to heart disease, and cerebral hemorrhage deaths exceeded those due to cerebral infarction.

In the United States, Kannel,[6] comparing epidemiologic features of brain infarction with myocardial infarction, investigated 5,106 men and women, age thirty to sixty-two, who at the outset of the study were found with no evidence of coronary heart disease or vascular disease of the brain. Over a period of twelve years, 167 myocardial infarctions and 57 thrombotic brain infarctions occurred. In men, the incidence of brain infarctions lagged twenty years behind myocardial infarctions. In 63 percent of the cases, the stroke was caused by cerebral thrombosis, as compared with only 4 percent by cerebral hemorrhage. Subarachnoid hemorrhage and cerebral embolism occurred in 15 percent.

According to Metropolitan Life Insurance Statistics,[7] one out of each nine deaths occurring in the United States is due to vascular lesions of the central nervous system, predominantly cerebral thrombosis, hemorrhage, and embolism. In addition to the deaths in which C.V.A.'s are mentioned as the primary cause, there are three fourths as many more in which C.V.A.'s are contributory causes. According to these same statistics, while the morbidity of C.V.A.'s is increasing, mostly because of the increasing aging population, the trend in mortality seems to be downward. For example, in 1952-53, the annual death rate per 100,000 was 86.7 for white males, and 78.6 for white females; ten years later, i.e. 1962-63, the death rate was reduced by 10 percent in males, and 16 percent in females to 77.6 and 66.6 per 100,000, respectively. A similar trend was seen in nonwhites, namely from 146.2 in males and 153.4 in females to 134.5 in males, and 131.8 in females, a reduction of 8 percent and 14 percent, respectively.

This is true of all age groups in whites until we reach the age of eighty-five and over. Here the mortality has increased, 28 percent among males and 43 percent among females. While some of these reductions may be a result of better care and treatment available in recent years, the reduction may also in part be because of a change in coding introduced in 1959 by the World Health Organization, which has suggested that some of these deaths be labeled as the result of heart disease because of the concomitant arteriosclerosis and hypertension.

What about those who survive and are not exposed to a proper rehabilitative program? Most of these are transferred to nursing homes. Let us briefly examine what happens to these stroke patients.

STROKE PATIENTS IN NURSING HOMES

The U.S. Department of Health, Education, and Welfare[8] reports on the prevalence of chronic conditions and impairments among residents of nursing and personal care homes. Of a total of 554,000 such residents, 188,100 were suffering from vascular lesions affecting the central nervous system. If we include those suffering from hypertension, 35,100, and those suffering from general arteriosclerosis, 43,500, we have a total of 266,700, or just about one-half the population in these homes. In addition are listed 66,600 as "palsy due to stroke." It can thus be seen that the number of residents suffering from cerebrovascular diseases in nursing homes total more than those suffering from all other causes combined. And what is even more serious is that a survey of these residents as to their mobility revealed the following: In the case of paralysis due to stroke, 249.7 residents out of 1,000 were limited to their beds, and 126.4 out of 1,000 were limited to their rooms. If we take the general group of "vascular diseases affecting the nervous system," 522.7 out of 1,000, that is over one-half the nursing home population, were limited to their beds or rooms. It would seem that many, if not most, of these unfortunate people were not exposed to a satisfactory rehabilitation program.

How many thousands, who have recovered from an acute stroke, are now at home, hibernating, can only be imagined.

Chapter 2

ETIOLOGY AND PATHOPHYSIOLOGY

STROKE POTENTIAL

T HE potential for developing C.V.A.'s may be judged from the fact that 40 percent of the population over fifty have intracranial or extracranial atherosclerosis to a degree which produces 50 percent stenosis of one or more major arteries.[9] It is estimated that 50 percent of these people will develop permanent neurologic lesions, and of all persons in this group who die, 20-25 percent have actual brain lesions resulting from vascular disease. Robinson[10] reviewed the records of 1,018 patients with diagnosis of cerebral thrombosis admitted to three hospitals in Worcester, Massachusetts, 1947 to 1965. The initial mortality was 21 percent. Of the survivors, 15 percent died within a year, and 60 percent died within five years. According to M. Fisher,[11] one out of ten men, women, and children living today has serious blockage of one or both cervical carotids. This may be present without symptoms, which occur only when the blood supply becomes inadequate because of cardiovascular or other conditions, to meet the demands of the brain.

ATHEROPOIESIS OR ATHEROGENESIS

Irving H. Page[12] postulates that atherogenesis is the same wherever the arteries occur. He discusses two theories: (a) *The filtration theory:* Lipids in blood plasma filter through the vessel wall into intracellular space, lymph, and back into circulation. Sometimes the lipids stick in the filter bed, and indissoluble lipid is freed and acts as a foreign body with resulting liberation of mucopolysaccharide, and scar and fibrous plaque formation. (b) *The encrustation theory:* Fibrin or platelets are laid down on normal endothelium. A cushion of cells is formed by the endothelium into which lipid may be deposited. With platelets, the thrombus is incorporated into the intima, followed by the appearance of lipids. Page believes that greater evidence points to the lipid infiltration concept of atherogenesis.

BRAIN TISSUE REQUIREMENTS

Brain tissues require an adequate blood flow for proper functioning. When the blood supply to a part of the brain is temporarily interrupted, we have a T.I.A. (transient ischemic attack). If the blood supply is quickly restored, then there is recovery from this T.I.A. If, on the other hand, the blood supply is interrupted for more than a few hours, we have an advancing stroke or a stroke in evolution. If the blood supply is interrupted permanently, then we have a completed stroke.

PATHOPHYSIOLOGY

Pathogenesis of a Completed Stroke

The pathogenesis of a completed stroke consists of the permanent interruption of the blood supply to a part of the brain. The causes of this interruption are (a) cerebral thrombosis, (b) cerebral hemorrhage, (c) cerebral embolism, and (d) rupture of a berry aneurism, which is really a modification of (b).

Cerebral Thrombosis

The underlying factor in cerebral thrombosis is atheromatosis. We mentioned above the two possible ways in which atheromatosis develops. But with either theory, the actual causes of the development of atheromatosis are hypertension and hypercholesteremia. However, once the atheromatosis has developed in a vessel, any further reduction in its lumen will result in thrombosis. The causes of such reduction are an increased size of atheromatous plaque, arteriolar spasm, polycythemia, neoplasm, and encephalitis. Step 1 is the deposition of blood platelets on the atheromatous plaque; step 2, reduced blood flow; step 3, blood clotting, and step 4, shutting off the lumen of a cerebral artery.

The degree of involvement depends on (a) the size of the clot, (b) its location, and (c) the amount of collateral circulation. If a small arteriole is involved, the damage may be slight. But when a major artery is closed by the clot and no collateral circulation develops, then we have brain infarction in the part supplied by the closed artery.

Cerebral Embolism

The pathophysiology of cerebral embolism is the same as for cerebral thrombosis, except that the clot reaches the brain from a distal part of the body, usually the heart.

Cerebral Hemorrhage

In cerebral hemorrhage, the arteriole ruptures, causing an escape of blood to the corresponding tissues with loss of nutrition and again resulting in infarction. Sometimes this is called hemorrhagic infarction.

Berry Aneurism

Berry aneurism, if ruptured, produces a similar effect as cerebral hemorrhage.

Infarct

A *cerebral infarct* is an area of ischemic necrosis resulting from prolonged cerebral hypoxia due to an arterial occlusion with inadequate collateral circulation.

Risk Factors

As already indicated, it is important for the stroke rehabilitation team to realize that when a stroke has once developed, no degree of treatment can guarantee its nonrecurrence as long as the risk factors which resulted in the stroke are still active. Therefore, we emphasize the risk factors which are as follows: (a) hypertension, (b) diabetes mellitus, (c) heart disease, (d) hypercholesteremia, (e) overweight, and (f) cigarette smoking.[13] A seventh risk factor is hyperthyroidism. The two salient keys to the production and prevention of stroke are hypertensive cardiovascular disease and atherosclerotic cardiovascular disease.

Other Causes of Diminished Blood Flow

Before concluding this chapter, we should mention other factors that may be responsible for the development of a stroke.[14] *Hypoxia* may be an important factor, since many of these patients

suffer from chronic bronchitis and emphysema. Continued cerebral hypoxia can cause intimal damage, even in the absence of
thrombosis or embolisms. *Lowering* of *blood pressure* may be
responsible for lowering of cerebral blood flow with resulting
T.I.A. (transient ischemic attack) or even a completed stroke.
Anemia may be a contributing factor. *Hemorrhage* from whatever cause may result in a C.V.A. if the other factors are present.
Vasospasm of the smaller vessels is not possible as the walls of
the smaller cerebral arterioles do not seem to have muscle or elastic
tissue. However, the larger extracranial arteries do have elastic
and muscle fibers. Therefore, spasm of these arteries is possible
with resulting stenosis. Given such stenosis, associated with hy-
potension or anemia, cerebral infarction is not only possible, but
likely.

A committee of the National Disease and Blindness of the National Institute of Health[15] has named more than fifty cerebrovascular diseases which can cause a stroke. The three primary
causes are (a) ischemia with or without subsequent cerebral
infarction (b) intracranial hemorrhage, and (c) cerebral embolism. According to J. F. Toole,[16] the pathogenesis of stroke
can be classified under two causes:

1. Interference with perfusion of brain tissue resulting in
   infarction.

2. Rupture of a vessel supplying the central nervous system
   with resulting destruction of nerve cells, directly by the
   blood, or later by the formed blood clot.

Summarizing, for proper functioning, the brain requires a satisfactory blood supply, ample hemoglobin, and adequate oxygenation. This means: (a) good circulation through the arteries
supplying the brain—common carotids, internal carotids, vertebral, basilar, circle of Willis, and the arterioles supplying all parts
of the brain; (b) adequate cardiac output, (c) adequate oxygen
in blood, and (d) adequate oxygenation of blood in the lungs.
Diminution of any of these requirements may be a predisposing
cause of stroke. This is what happens so often in the older age
group.

SUMMARY

In the preceding paragraphs, I have indicated the general view of the etiology and pathophysiology of stroke. I should like to end this chapter with some thoughts that I have developed on this subject. There is great to-do about trying to find the stroke-prone patient with a view to preventing strokes. This is well and should be continued. But all of us have seen repeatedly in well-run hospitals, patients who have had one, or two, or more strokes, develop a stroke while in the hospital and under the best possible care. It is obvious that a patient who has had one or two strokes is a stroke-prone individual. Yet, in spite of all our care, he or she still develops another stroke. So it is not enough to find the stroke-prone individual. What is even more important is to find out how to prevent the occurrence of another stroke. Furthermore, all the theories of stroke development fail to emphasize what seems to me to be a very important observation. We see many couples married for thirty or more years, eating the same food, living in the same environment. Yet, the husband or wife will develop a stroke, while the partner does not seem to be affected. It would seem obvious that some hereditary or early childhood influence plays an important part in such stroke-prone individuals. If this is so, then should we not better begin with the study of the genetics, as well as habits of early childhood, to see if we can prevent the development of the bases for cerebrovascular accident in later years?

Chapter 3

EVALUATION

W HEN a patient has been admitted to the hospital with apparent symptoms of a stroke, the ward physician or his personal physician takes a careful history from him and his family, does a routine physical examination, orders appropriate x-ray and laboratory tests, makes a tentative diagnosis, and calls in necessary consultants for more expert evaluation. Based upon these examinations and tests, a diagnosis is made of a C.V.A. An attempt is made at the localization and type of lesion, and the indicated definitive treatment is instituted. Consistent with good modern practice, the physician then calls in consultation a physiatrist, if available, or if a qualified physiatrist is not available, he calls in a physician interested in physical medicine and rehabilitation. The physiatrist consultant goes to the patient's bedside, if necessary, or calls for the patient to come to the PM&R (physical medicine and rehabilitation) clinic with his chart, if the patient can be moved, and makes an evaluation from the PM&R standpoint and prescribes the appropriate PM&R procedures.

The appropriate procedures, based upon the PM&R findings will be discussed in succeeding chapters. At this time we shall describe the various evaluations pertinent to prescribing a proper rehabilitation routine. These evaluations include some or all of the following, as indicated: a neurological survey, a motor functional evaluation, a sensory evaluation, and an A.D.L. (activities of daily living) evaluation. We shall now discuss each in turn.

NEUROLOGICAL SURVEY

Usually a neurologist has made a thorough neurological examination, but it behooves the physiatrist to review this examination, and if necessary, to confirm some of these findings. A check list for such a neurological examination published in connection with the film "Essentials of the Neurological Examination"[17] includes tests for cerebral function, tests for cranial nerves, tests for cerebellar function, tests for the motor system, tests for the sensory system, and tests for reflex status. A booklet, a movie, and a checklist are available for this purpose.

This neurological survey helps to categorize the type and degree of lesion. For the purpose of instituting a P.M. and R. program, it needs to be supplemented by the additional tests above mentioned. Based upon the results of these tests, the physiatrist then prescribes appropriate procedures to be administered by the rest of the rehabilitation team. The various objectives of these procedures are to relieve pain, if present, to promote function, to restore mobility, to prevent contractures, to improve coordination, to assist with developing communications, to relieve anxiety in the patient and family, and finally, to set a rehabilitation goal for the patient. The rehabilitation goal for the patient will depend upon the results of such evaluations. We shall now proceed to describe these evaluations.

STROKE MOTOR FUNCTION EVALUATION

It is necessary to understand that at the onset of a cerebrovascular accident, the average patient will be too sick and too weak for us to conduct the examination that follows. Only when he is apparently out of danger and ready for an intensive rehabilitation program is such functional evaluation meaningful. While many physiatrists have developed extensive functional evaluation routines, e.g., Dinken,[18] Deaver,[19] Thomas,[20,21] Institute of Crippled and Disabled,[22] and Rusk,[23] I believe that the Hemiplegia Motor Function Evaluation form developed by the Department of Medicine and Surgery of the U.S. Veterans Administration is the simplest and most useful (Fig. 1). The reader will note that these are all tests of motor function and not tests of individual muscle strength, such as are used in peripheral paralysis, as, for example, in poliomyelitis. The reason for this is that in peripheral paralysis there is weakness or paralysis of all muscles supplied by a certain nerve, or by a certain nerve root. This paralysis or weakness can be graded from zero to normal. This is not true in patients with stroke paralysis. The spastic quadriceps, for example, involved in

CLINICAL RECORD	HEMIPLEGIA MOTOR FUNCTION EVALUATION						
DIAGNOSIS AND BRIEF CLINICAL HISTORY							

NOTE. - At no time does the examiner touch the patient. Whatever angles or distances are involved, record actual values in degrees or inches. These measurements are to be taken only on active movement. KEY for evaluating functions is on the reverse side.

		EXAMINER'S INITIALS					REMARKS
		DATE					
HEAD-NECK (Standing in Parallel Bars)	EXTENSION						
	BEND RIGHT						
	BEND LEFT						
	ROTATE RIGHT						
	ROTATE LEFT						
UPPER EXTREMITY (Sitting)	RAISE ARM OVERHEAD						
	HAND TO MOUTH						
	HAND BEHIND BACK						
	FORWARD REACH						
	TURN PALM UP						
	TURN PALM DOWN						
	GRASP						
	GRASP AND RELEASE						
	OPEN HAND						
	PINCH AND RELEASE						
TRUNK (Sitting)	ARMS AT SIDES, BEND TO RIGHT						
	ARMS AT SIDES, BEND TO LEFT						
	ARMS FOLDED, TWIST TO RIGHT						
	ARMS FOLDED, TWIST TO LEFT						
	ARMS FOLDED, LEAN FORWARD AND RETURN						
LOWER EXTREMITY (Standing in Parallel Bars)	BEND KNEE AND RAISE LEG						
	LEFT LEG - PLACE DOWN HEEL FIRST						
	RAISE LEG TO SIDE						
	RAISE GOOD LEG						
	BEND INVOLVED KNEE; RAISE GOOD LEG						
AMBULATION DEFICITS (Standing in Parallel Bars)	LOSS OF BALANCE: DIRECTION:						
	HIP DROP						
	GENU RECURVATUM						
	TOE DRAG						
	SUPINATION OF FOOT						
	HIP ADDUCTION						
OTHER (List)							

PATIENT'S LAST NAME, FIRST NAME, MIDDLE INITIAL: IDENTIFICATION NO.: WARD NO.: NAME OF STATION

CLINICAL RECORD
HEMIPLEGIA MOTOR FUNCTION EVALUATION

Figure 1. Hemiplegia Motor Function Evaluation Form. a. *(this page)* Front.

stroke paralysis, which might be graded "poor" in the supine position, will, when the patient stands, be able to support his weight. Or the iliopsoas which might be "poor" during bed rest will, when the patient walks, be able to flex his hip during the swing phase of ambulation.

The Hemiplegia Motor Function Evaluation that follows, tests

HEMIPLEGIA MOTOR FUNCTION EVALUATION *(Continued)*							
TAKEN IN A SITTING POSITION	EXAMINER'S INITIALS ▶						**REMARKS**
	DATE ▶						
HAND TO MOUTH, SUPINATE FOREARM	GRASP AND RELEASE						
	OPEN HAND						
	PINCH AND RELEASE						
HAND TO MOUTH, PRONATE FOREARM	GRASP AND RELEASE						
	OPEN HAND						
	PINCH AND RELEASE						
FORWARD REACH, PRONATE FOREARM	GRASP AND RELEASE						
	OPEN HAND						
	PINCH AND RELEASE						
FORWARD REACH, SUPINATE FOREARM	GRASP AND RELEASE						
	OPEN HAND						
	PINCH AND RELEASE						
RAISE ARM OVERHEAD, PRONATE FOREARM	GRASP AND RELEASE						
	OPEN HAND						
	PINCH AND RELEASE						
RAISE ARM OVERHEAD, SUPINATE FOREARM	GRASP AND RELEASE						
	OPEN HAND						
	PINCH AND RELEASE						
HAND BEHIND BACK, PRONATE FOREARM	GRASP AND RELEASE						
	OPEN HAND						
	PINCH AND RELEASE						
HAND BEHNIND BACK, SUPINATE FOREARM	GRASP AND RELEASE						
	OPEN HAND						
	PINCH AND RELEASE						
	GRASP AND RELEASE						
	OPEN HAND						
	PINCH AND RELEASE						

REMARKS

PHYSICIAN'S SIGNATURE — DATE

KEY:

HEAD - NECK, UPPER EXTREMITY	TRUNK, LOWER EXTREMITY	AMBULATION DEFICITS
G - Good completion of motion	SY - Spasticity	G - Good no deficits
Pt - Partial, completion of motion	Sm - Spasm	Mn - Minimal deficits
Mn - Minimal amount of motion	C - Contracture	Md - Moderate deficits
O - Zero motion performed	P - Pain	Mk - Marked deficits

Figure 1b. Hemiphlegia Motor Function Evaluation Form. Back.

the patient both during sitting and standing. When the patient is able to accomplish a motion, the date is recorded on the form. Thus the physician and the rest of the rehabilitation team can, at a glance, note the patient's progress.

The test is divided into fourteen sections and graded for two groups: (a) head, neck, and upper extremity, and (b) trunk, lower extremity; with grades of *G*—good when the motion is completed, *Pt*—partial when the motion is not completed, *mn*—minimal motion, and *O*—no motion; *SY*—spasticity, *Sm*—spasm, *C*—contracture, and *P*—pain.

Ambulation deficits are noted: *Good*—no deficits, *Mn*—minimal deficits, *Md*—moderate deficits, and *Mk*—marked deficits, patient can walk, but with great difficulty. Room is provided on the chart for "Others" and for "Remarks."

The tests are as follows (note—the examiner does not touch the patient):

Head-Neck (patient standing in parallel bars): patient is asked to bend head back (extension), and bend it right, and left; turn (rotate) right and left.

Upper Extremity (sitting): patient is asked to raise paretic arm over head; place hand to mouth; put hand behind back; reach forward; turn palm up; turn palm down; grasp an object and release; open hand; pinch an object and release.

Trunk (sitting): arms at sides, bend to right, bend to left; arms folded, twist to right, twist to left; arms folded, lean forward and return.

Lower Extremity (standing between parallel bars): bend knee and raise paretic leg; raise paretic leg, put it down, heel first; raise paretic leg sideways; stand on paretic leg and raise nonparetic leg; bend the paretic knee, stand on paretic leg, and raise nonparetic leg.

Ambulation Deficits (patient standing between paralled bars): take hands off bars, watch for loss of balance, note direction; watch for hip drop; look for genu recurvatum; observe toe drag; note foot supination; note hip adduction.

Other, list any deficit previously not noted, e.g. is patient inclined to lean backwards, is there clonus? Is the patient inclined to "black out?"

Now the paretic upper extremity is further tested in sitting position.

Hand to mouth—supinate forearm, now grasp and release; open
hand, pinch and release.

Hand to mouth—pronate forearm, repeat as above.

Forward reach—forearm pronated, repeat as above.

Forward reach—forearm supinated, repeat as above.

Raise arm overhead—pronate forearm, repeat as above.

Raise arm overhead—supinate forearm, repeat as above.

Hand behind back—pronate forearm, repeat as above.

Hand behind back—supinate forearm, repeat as above.

In blank column we can add:

*Hand far out at side—*pronate and supinate forearm, grasp and
release, open hand, pinch and release.

SENSORY EVALUATION

The third type of evaluation is the sensory evaluation. To examine for sensation disturbances, later considered in the chapter
on dysesthesia, the Veterans Administration has developed a sensory examination form (VA Form 531, Sensory Examination—
Superficial and Deep). (Fig. 2 shows a modified version of this
form). The form is divided into quarters: Touch, Pain, Tempera-
ture, and Position—Vibration. The testing is done in the usual
manner, and the areas of anesthesia, analgesia, athermia, and
pallanesthesia are indicated on the form, either as total absence,
or partial disturbance, as the case may be. In the chapter on
dysesthesia, we shall describe a more accurate method of mapping
out areas of pallhypesthesia and pallanesthesia.

A.D.L. (ACTIVITIES OF DAILY LIVING)

Finally, it is often necessary to test a patient for the activities of
daily living, or as we often shorten the term, A.D.L. This test is
especially indicated in stroke patients who will not become pro-
ficient at independent ambulation, but will reach a less satisfactory phase in their rehabilitation, such as bed phase, dependent
wheelchair, or independent wheelchair phase, or even dependent
ambulation phase. In such cases, it is necessary to assess their
A.D.L. capabilities and to teach them, as much as possible, in
view of their disability, to take care of their daily needs. The emphasis is on one-handed activities.

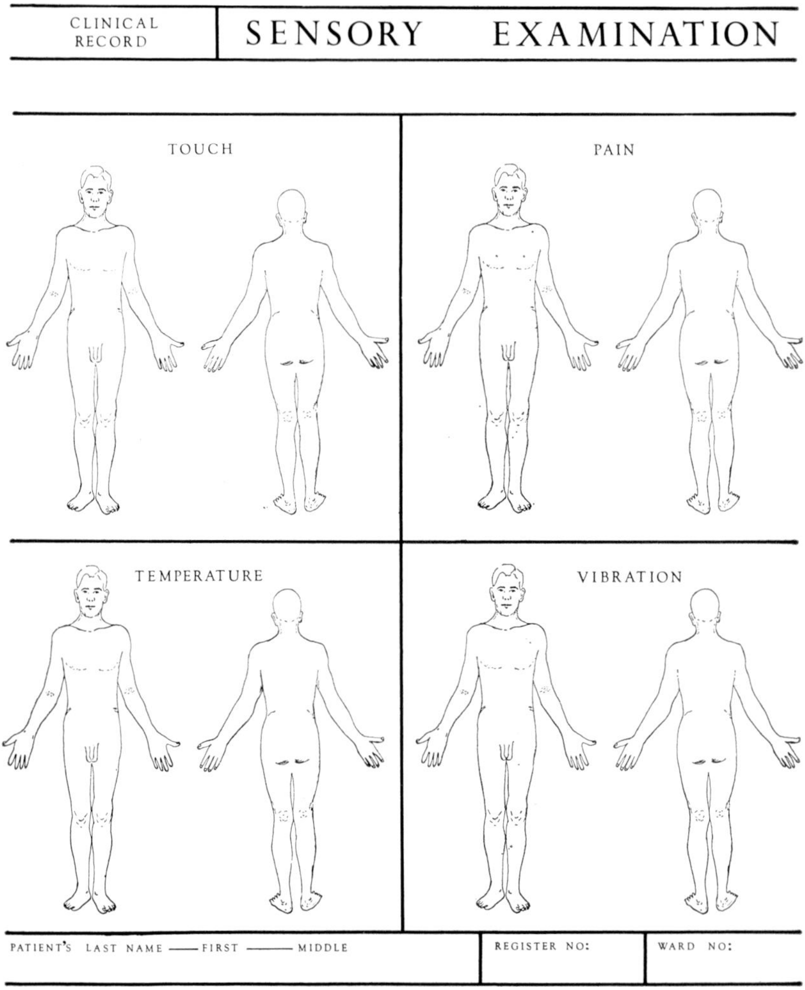

CLINICAL RECORD	SENSORY EXAMINATION

Figure 2. Modified Sensory Examination Form. Sensory examination, superficial and deep.

For this purpose there has been produced by the Veterans Administration a fairly complete form which is called Self-care Activities—Functional Evaluation (VA Form 10-2617) (Fig. 3). This form consists of eight parts. Each part is subdivided into various categories. The completion of this form will give the members of the rehabilitation team an excellent idea of the capabilities of their patients.

Briefly, this form is subdivided into seven headings, each with

CLINICAL RECORD	SELF-CARE ACTIVITIES—FUNCTIONAL EVALUATION

TYPE OF DISABILITY

PRECAUTIONS

HANDEDNESS ☐ LEFT ☐ RIGHT	ORTHOPEDIC APPLIANCE(S)	OCCUPATION (*Prehospitalization*)	AGE

INITIAL TEST		SCORING KEY
THERAPIST INITIALS	THERAPIST INITIALS	(*Scores indicate skill accomplished within a reasonable time*) 0—Cannot be accomplished. 1—Can be accomplished with human aid. 2—Can be accomplished with adaptation of environment (low bed, special toilet seat, hand rails, ramps, etc.). 3—Can be accomplished with use of mechanical aids (splints, braces, prostheses, crutches, wheelchair, etc.). 4—Can be accomplished without aids, adaptation or assistance.
DATE INITIAL TEST COMPLETED		

ACTIVITIES	SCORE (*RED X—indicates initial test; DATE—indicates change in condition*)				
PART I—EATING	0	1	2	3	4
1. EAT WITH FINGERS					
2. DRINK FROM CUP					
3. DRINK FROM GLASS					
4. EAT WITH SPOON					
5. CUT WITH KNIFE					
6. CUT WITH FORK					
7. EAT WITH FORK					
8. MAINTAIN SUITABLE POSTURE					
9.					
10.					
11.					
PART II—COMMUNICATION					
12. WRITE					
13. TYPE					
14. USE TELEPHONE					
15. OPEN ENVELOPE					
16. REMOVE LETTER FROM ENVELOPE					
17. PLACE LETTER IN ENVELOPE AND SEAL					
18.					
19.					
20.					
PART III—HYGIENE					
21. TURN ON FAUCET					
22. TURN OFF FAUCET					
23. SHAVE					
24. MAKE UP					
25. WASH HANDS					
26. WASH FACE					
27. BRUSH OR COMB HAIR					
28. SHAMPOO HAIR					
29. BRUSH TEETH					

SIGNATURE OF CHIEF, PHYSICAL MEDICINE AND REHABILITATION	DATE

PATIENT'S LAST NAME—FIRST NAME—MIDDLE NAME	REGISTER NO.	WARD NO.

NAME OF HOSPITAL OR OTHER MEDICAL FACILITY	SELF-CARE ACTIVITIES—FUNCTIONAL EVALUATION

Figure 3. Self-care Activities—Functional Evaluation. a. (*this page*) Part I—Eating, Part II—Communication, Part III—Hygiene.

ACTIVITIES	SCORE (RED X—indicates initial test; DATE—indicates change in condition)				
	0	1	2	3	4
PART III—HYGIENE (Continued)					
30. GET INTO BATH					
31. GET OUT OF BATH					
32. GET INTO SHOWER					
33. GET OUT OF SHOWER					
34. BATHE SELF					
35. USE URINAL					
36. USE BEDPAN					
37. GET ON TOILET					
38. ADJUST CLOTHING					
39. GET OFF TOILET					
40. READJUST CLOTHING					
41. TRIM FINGERNAILS					
42. CLEAN FINGERNAILS					
43. TRIM TOENAILS					
44. CLEAN TOENAILS					
45.					
46.					
47.					
PART IV—DRESSING					
48. PUT ON BRACES OR PROSTHESES					
49. REMOVE BRACES OR PROSTHESES					
50. PUT ON TROUSERS OR SKIRT					
51. REMOVE TROUSERS OR SKIRT					
52. PUT ON PULLOVER GARMENT					
53. REMOVE PULLOVER GARMENT					
54. PUT ON SHIRT OR BLOUSE					
55. REMOVE SHIRT OR BLOUSE					
56. BUTTON BUTTONS					
57. UNBUTTON BUTTONS					
58. ZIP ZIPPER					
59. UNZIP ZIPPER					
60. OPERATE HOOKS AND EYES					
61. SNAP SNAPS					
62. UNSNAP SNAPS					
63. PUT ON TIE SHOE OR BUCKLE SHOE					
64. REMOVE TIE SHOE OR BUCKLE SHOE					
65. TIE BOW					
66. UNTIE BOW					
67. BUCKLE BUCKLE					
68. UNBUCKLE BUCKLE					
69. PUT ON SLIPPERS OR LOAFERS					
70. REMOVE SLIPPERS OR LOAFERS					
71. PUT ON HOSE					
72. REMOVE HOSE					
73. PUT ON NECKTIE					
74. REMOVE NECKTIE					
75. PUT OBJECT IN POCKET					
76. REMOVE OBJECT FROM POCKET					
77.					
78.					
79.					
PART V—LOCOMOTION					
80. MOVE FROM PLACE TO PLACE IN BED					
81. TURN OVER IN BED					

Figure 3b. Part III—Hygiene (cont.), Part IV—Dressing, Part V—Locomotion.

subheadings as follows: Part I, Eating; eight specific subheadings, and three for additional remarks. Part II, Communication; six subheadings, and three for remarks. Part III, Hygiene; twenty-four subheadings, and three for additional remarks. Part IV, dressing, twenty-nine subheadings, and three for additional remarks. Part V, Locomotion; thirty-nine subheadings and three for additional remarks. Part VI, Household; eleven subheadings. Fin-

ACTIVITIES	SCORE (RED X—indicates initial test; DATE—indicates change in condition)				
PART V—LOCOMOTION (Continued)	0	1	2	3	4
82. SIT UP IN BED					
83. GET OUT OF BED TO CHAIR					
84. GET INTO BED FROM CHAIR					
85. GET OUT OF BED TO STANDING					
86. GET INTO BED FROM STANDING					
87. PROPEL WHEELCHAIR					
88. CHAIR TO STANDING					
89. STANDING TO CHAIR					
90. STAND					
91. STAND AND REMAIN IN ERECT POSITION					
92. WALK ON SMOOTH SURFACE— FT.					
93. WALK BACKWARD					
94. WALK SIDEWARD TO LEFT					
95. WALK SIDEWARD TO RIGHT					
96. WALK ON ROUGH SURFACES INCLUDING RUGS					
97. WALK UP RAMP— FT.					
98. WALK DOWN RAMP— FT.					
99. GO UP FLIGHT STAIRS					
100. GO DOWN FLIGHT STAIRS					
101. GO DOWN CURB					
102. GO UP CURB					
103. GO DOWN CURB—CROSS STREET—GO UP CURB					
104. OPEN DOOR—GO THROUGH—CLOSE DOOR					
105. GET DOWN TO FLOOR					
106. GET UP FROM FLOOR					
107. MOVE ON FLOOR IN OTHER THAN UPRIGHT POSITION					
108. GO UP BUS STEPS					
109. GO DOWN BUS STEPS					
110. GET INTO AUTOMOBILE					
111. GET OUT OF AUTOMOBILE					
112. DRIVE AUTOMOBILE					
113. WALK CARRYING TRAY WITH DISHES					
114. PLACE TRAY ON TABLE					
115. GET INTO CHURCH PEW					
116. GET OUT OF CHURCH PEW					
117. GET INTO THEATER SEAT					
118. GET OUT OF THEATER SEAT					
119.					
120.					
121.					
PART VI—HOUSEHOLD					
122. OPEN DRAWERS					
123. CLOSE DRAWERS					
124. LOCK DOOR					
125. UNLOCK DOOR					
126. GET INTO CHAIR AT TABLE					
127. GET OUT OF CHAIR AT TABLE					
128. GET INTO UPHOLSTERED CHAIR					
129. GET OUT OF UPHOLSTERED CHAIR					
130. MAKE BED					
131. OPEN WINDOW					
132. CLOSE WINDOW					
133.					
134.					

Figure 3c. Part V—Locomotion (cont.), Part VI—Household.

ally, Part VII, Miscellaneous; twenty subheadings. This A.D.L. examination is, of course, time consuming but thorough. Where there are sufficient personnel, it presents a real assessment of the patient's abilities. But it does take a great deal of time. Where

ACTIVITIES	SCORE (RED X—indicates initial test; DATE—indicates change in condition)				
PART VII—MISCELLANEOUS	0	1	2	3	4
135. USE PULL CORD					
136. USE PUSH BUTTONS					
137. USE TWIST KNOB					
138. WIND WATCH					
139. HOLD BOOK					
140. TURN PAGES					
141. HOLD NEWSPAPER					
142. TURN PAGES					
143. PICK UP OBJECT FROM TABLE					
144. PICK UP OBJECT FROM FLOOR					
145. HANDLE MONEY					
146. LIGHT CIGARETTE					
147. LIGHT PIPE					
148. TAKE GLASSES FROM POCKET OR CASE					
149. PUT GLASSES ON					
150. REPLACE GLASSES IN POCKET OR CASE					
151. USE NEEDLE AND THREAD					
152. OPEN SAFETY PIN					
153. PIN CLOTH					
154. CLOSE SAFETY PIN					
155.					
156.					
157.					
158.					
159.					
REMARKS					

Figure 3d. Part VII—Miscellaneous.

there is a small number of personnel, or where time is an important factor, I have prepared a simplified A.D.L. form (Fig. 4) which is divided into two main sections, namely Self-care and Ambulation. We have found that this form is adequate for most of our needs, as it can be accomplished with the average stroke

CLINICAL RECORD	Report on _____ or Continuation of S. F. _____ (Strike out one line)	PHYSICAL MEDICINE & REHAB. - ADL TEST (Specify type of examination or data)

SELF-CARE		(Sign and date)	AMBULATION	
Activity	Date*		Activity	Date*
1. Change position in bed			1. Chair to stand with aid in parallel bars	
2. Feed self				
3. Wash hands and face			2. Chair to stand without aid in parallel bars	
4. Brush teeth and comb hair				
5. Shave self			3. Walk in parallel bars with aid	
6. Write name			4. Walk in parallel bars without aid	
7. Sit up for six hours daily				
8. Get from lying position to sitting position.			5. Walk with aid of instructor	
			6. Walk with instructor by side	
9. Perform chair or wheelchair transfers			7. Stand from wheelchair without aid	
10. From sit on bed to stand			8. Walk with cane, crutch or crutches	
11. Propel wheelchair				
12. Use toilet without assistance			9. Go up and downstairs using handrail, cane or crutches	
13. Put on and remove pajama top				
14. Put on and remove pajama bottom			10. Go up and down stairs without using handrail, crutch or crutches	
15. Put on and remove shoes				
16. Bathe self			11. Walk sidewards and backwards	
17. Put on and remove brace			12. Walk up and down ramps	
18. Pick up object from floor			13. Walk on ground	
19. Use telephone			14. Open and close doors	
20. Get in and out of car			15. Go up and down curbs	
21. Get down to and up from floor			16. Walk 50 yards	
			17. Walk 15 yards in 1 minute (traffic light)	
* Indicates date activity can be accomplished.			18. Walk 100 yards in 5 minutes	

Date Initial Test Completed _____

_____ Therapist

O Indicates activity does not apply

(Continue on reverse side) HARRY T. ZANKEL, M.D.
Chief, PM&R Service

PATIENT'S IDENTIFICATION (For typed or written entries give: Name—last, first, middle; grade; date; hospital or medical facility)	REGISTER NO.	WARD NO.

REPORT ON _____ or CONTINUATION OF _____

Figure 4. Self-care and ambulation—A.D.L. Test.

patients in less than thirty minutes. Many of the answers can be received from the ward personnel. A date column next to the activity is filled in, when the patient can accomplish the activity. With the help of this form, we can assess the patient's needs and aim for his fulfillment.

Many other forms have been developed for evaluating self-care activities. I mention here a very complete form, which numerically measures the self-care abilities of patients. It is called the Numerical Scoring of Self-care Status of Patients, encompassing eighteen individual self-care items, each rated on a five points scale.[24] It would be very helpful to those studying A.D.L. from a research standpoint.

Chapter 4

GENERAL PRINCIPLES OF STROKE
REHABILITATION

THE following general principles of stroke rehabilitation will serve as a guide to the stroke rehabilitation team. Most of these are well known, but some are not adequately applied.

1. There is no question but that the earlier rehabilitation procedures are instituted, the better chance for functional recovery. Therefore, range of motion exercises should be instituted as soon as the patient has been admitted and the diagnosis made.
2. The younger the patient, the better chance for successful rehabilitation. Therefore, the younger patient calls for a more dynamic program. The older patient requires a more protective program.
3. A muscle that is not used atrophies. This will be discussed in Chapter 7 under "Prolonged Bed Rest—Deleterious Effects."
4. Paralyzed muscles need to be supported and protected against overstretching. Otherwise, the strong pull of the nonparetic muscles will produce flexion contractures.
5. A tendon or muscle that is allowed to shorten for a period of time tends to remain shortened.
6. The same is true of a joint, namely if allowed to contract, it tends to remain contracted.
7. Habit patterns, once developed, are difficult to break. This does not mean that a seventy-year-old stroke patient should be forced to learn a so-called correct gait. It does mean that we should try and teach every stroke patient the proper gait that is best for his purposes.
8. Reeducation is enhanced by repetition. The idea of walking with a stroke patient one-half hour daily is not consid-

ered adequate by this rule. It is better to get the patient out of bed and out of the wheelchair, if possible, and help him walk, five to ten minutes out of every hour, or even more often.

9. For an adequate stroke rehabilitation program, one does not need full-time professional personnel to be with the patient at all times. Properly trained subprofessional personnel, volunteers, or family, under professional guidance, can be just as helpful.

10. We should get away from using the word "normal" when we speak of the nonparetic extremity. The same is true of the word "uninvolved."

    a. Eighty-five percent of the limb muscles are supplied by the contralateral side of the brain; 15 percent from the same side.[25] Therefore, in left hemiplegia, the right lower extremity is not normal, but 15 percent below normal.

    b. The nonparetic extremity frequently shows abnormal electromyographic patterns.[26]

11. Sensory stimulation properly applied will facilitate or inhibit motor response at the proper spinal level.

12. Sherrington's Law of Reciprocal Innervations: Stimulation of agonist causes relaxation of antagonists. This is applied in the S.A.E. routine (Chapter 12).

13. As brought out in our introduction and definition of a stroke, the results obtained in an experimental animal by ablation of a part of the brain, while interesting and helpful, cannot be expected to apply to a stroke patient, who has localized brain damage in a brain, involved in an atherosclerotic process.

14. It is conceded that some patients, with a mild C.V.A., will recover without any rehabilitation effort. However, most patients will require such assistance and should be given the benefit of it.

15. Finally, in a patient following a stroke, it is important to determine not only the degree of involvement, but also the degree of disability and the potential for recovery. This is done by early and repeated evaluations. These we have considered in the previous chapter.

Chapter 5

EARLY CARE

WHILE a more complete description of the stroke rehabilitation routine will be given under the various phases of Part II, we shall now describe the management of a patient in the very beginning of his hospitalization. This is done so that all the necessary measures can be grouped together because of their importance in the early care of a stroke patient.

Immediately following a stroke, the patient manifests a variable degree of unconsciousness. There is flaccid paralysis of all extremities, bladder, and rectum. The patient is more or less helpless. While the physician proceeds with the indicated diagnostic and therapeutic measures to save life, the members of the rehabilitation team also have a very important function to perform even during this bed phase. Attention should be given by the members of the team to the details which follow.

WITH THE PATIENT UNCONSCIOUS OR SEMICONSCIOUS

1. The *bed* should be high or Hi-low® so that the doctor, the nurse, nurse's aid, and therapist can perform their functions with utmost efficiency (Fig. 5a, b).

2. *Side rails* should be provided, so that the patient can not fall out of bed (Fig. 6).

3. If necessary, the patient's upper and lower extremities *should be tied to the bed,* but loosely, to prevent him from rolling over the side rails.

4. A *foot board* should be placed at the foot of the bed and the patient's feet held at a 90-degree angle, while he is in a supine position. A blanket support at foot of bed keeps pressure off feet (Fig. 7).

5. The patient should be *turned every hour* from supine, to side

29

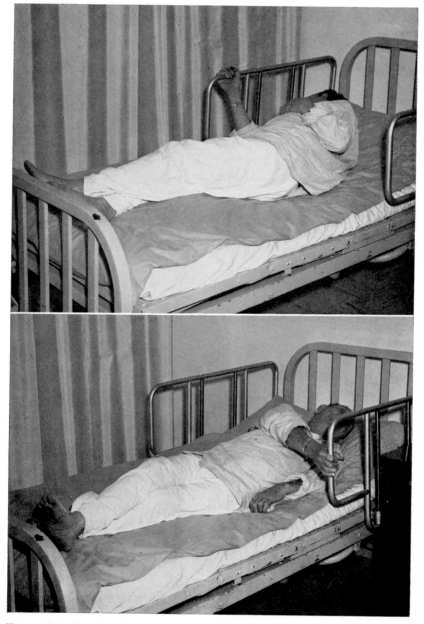

Figure 5. Bed with side rails. a. *(top)* Left hemiplegic patient lying on right side. b. *(bottom)* Patient has used side-rail to turn to left side.

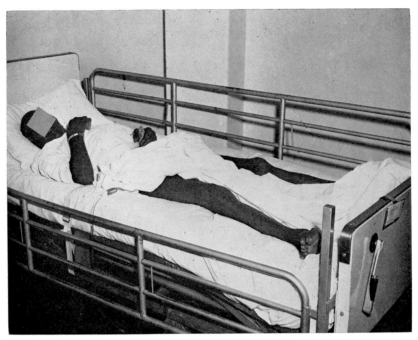

Figure 6. Hi-low bed for stroke patient. Note hand roll in each hand to prevent flexion contracture of fingers.

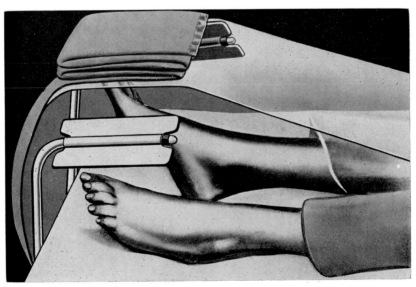

Figure 7. Blanket support at foot of bed to keep pressure off feet.

positions, first one side, then the other, but he should not be allowed to lie too long on the paretic side.

6. When in supine position, a *sand bag* should be placed at side of paralyzed foot to keep it from everting.

7. A *pillow* should be placed between arm and chest to prevent adduction.

8. *An alternate method* is to place the paretic upper extremity in the Statue of Liberty position, at regular intervals, i.e., fifteen minutes out of every hour, alternating with pillow position.

9. *Bladder* should be emptied at regular intervals by physician, nurse, or qualified aide by catheterization, under aseptic precautions. We do not believe in inserting a permanent indwelling catheter unless the patient is unconscious more than forty eight hours, as the danger of infection is greater from continuous catheterizations than it is from intermittent catheterizations. However, if sufficient help is not available and a permanent indwelling catheter is inserted, it should be opened at regular intervals, and the bladder should be irrigated with an antiseptic solution, such as Suby's solution G, which helps to dissove calcium phosphate and calcium carbonate calculi, as well as prevent urinary tract infection.

10. *Bowels* should be emptied by enema until return is clear. Repeat every forty eight hours if necessary.

11. *Paralysis.* Since at this stage the patient is unable to exercise his extremities, these should be put through passive range of motion at least twice a day. This can be done by the therapist, nurse, or aide. Chapter 7 will give details of these exercises.

The above program should be repeated as long as the patient is unconscious.

RETURN OF CONSCIOUSNESS

Within a variable period, depending on the cause of the stroke and the degree of brain damage, the patient will gradually, or sometimes, suddenly, return to consciousness. When this occurs, the program will be changed to the following.

1. *Patient Orientation.* The doctor should assure the patient,

and the other members of the team should, by their actions, confirm this assurance that, if the patient cooperates, his chances for a satisfactory rehabilitation result are good. This is done even if the patient is dysphasic, and not, immediately, responsive to direction, on the assumption that he understands what is said.

2. *Family Orientation.* Reassure the family that now that the patient has regained consciousness, his prognosis is much better. Explain to them that the fact that he is aphasic does not mean that he has lost his mind. Point out to them that their attitude is very important, not only to the patient, but to the other members of the rehabilitation team. An attitude of hopefulness will tend to create a similar attitude in the patient, while an attitude of helplessness or negativism will tend to create a corresponding effect on the patient. The patient should be made to feel that he is wanted, and he will make a better effort toward his recovery, assuming, of course, that his mentation is satisfactory, as will be pointed out in a later chapter. (See Chapter 17, "Dysmentia.)"

3. *Mobility.* As soon as his condition warrants, whether this is the second day or any subsequent day, have the patient sit up in bed with his feet hanging over the edge of the bed. If he reacts satisfactorily, then have him stand, with your help, a few minutes every hour.

4. *Exercise.* The therapist and nursing staff continue to give the patient passive exercise to the paretic extremities and remind the patient to do active exercises with the nonparetic limbs. Furthermore, they encourage the patient to exercise the paretic extremities by means of the nonparetic extremities, using the nonparetic hand to exercise the paretic upper extremity, and the nonparetic ankle and foot to lift and move the paretic lower extremity. An overhead pulley installed over the head of the bed will be of help in this regard. Between exercises, a hand roll or splint is placed, respectively, in or on paretic hand to prevent flexion contractures of fingers.

5. *Bladder.* As soon as the patient is able to stand, the catheter, if it has been inserted, is removed, and the patient is offered a urinal at regular intervals for voiding at the bedside, if

necessary. If the patient cannot void and recatheterization is necessary, then a second effort should be made in a few hours and should be repeated even a third or fourth time in the hope that spontaneous voiding will develop.

6. *Bowels.* When the patient is able to stand, he should be encouraged to move his bowels, at the bedside commode if necessary, or, preferably, he should be assisted to the lavatory for this purpose. Here it is important to know the patient's prestroke bowel habits and to apply them. For example, if the patient has been in the habit of reading a newspaper or magazine, this procedure should be followed. If, in the past, he has required some prune juice, this should be given to him. If he has been accustomed to a fecal softener, such as a Surfak,® this should be administered. Laxatives should be avoided unless the patient has been accustomed to them, in which case a bowel training program should be instituted as soon as possible. (See "Bowel and Bladder Training," Chapter 21.)

7. *Self-Care.* As soon as the patient has regained the use of his nonparetic upper extremity, encourage simple self-care activities, such as self-feeding, shaving with an electric razor, combing his hair, brushing his teeth, and moving about the bed using the nonparetic limbs to assist the paretic ones. For patients whose paretic upper extremity remains functionless, one-handed activties are encouraged. (See Chapter 23.)

At this time, if the patient has been in a Hi-low® bed, it should be lowered, or if he has been in a high bed, he should be moved to a low bed, for easier transfer from bed to chair and vice versa.

The above instructions form a general outline of the care of a patient in the early stages of his stroke. In the following chapters, we shall describe some of these procedures in greater detail.

PART II
THE STROKE 4-DYS SYNDROME

INTRODUCTION

When we speak of a stroke, we usually think of a left hemiplegia or a right hemiplegia and aphasia. We are apt to forget that there is more to a cerebrovascular accident than paralysis and loss of communication. It is therefore advisable to consider a stroke as a four-pronged syndrome: (a) disturbed motor function, (b) disturbed sensory function, (c) disturbed communication, and (d) disturbed mentation. We have given the names to these symptom groups as (a) Dyskinesia, (b) Dysesthesia, (c) Dysphasia, and (d) Dysmentia. Each of these and its ramification will be discussed separately as to manifestations and management.

Chapter 6

DYSKINESIA

W HEN we say *hemiplegia,* we mean *paralysis,* if there is complete loss of motor power, or *paresis* if there is partial loss of motor power. But this loss of motor power represents only a part of the disturbed motor function. For in addition to loss of motor power, there usually is an associated spasticity and sometimes incoordination. I, therefore, prefer to use the term *dyskinesia* as applicable to all these manifestations. *Dys-kinesia* is derived from the Greek *dys* meaning disturbance of, and *kineo,* meaning motion. Dyskinesia then, is manifested by the following: (a) paralysis, or total loss of motor power; or paresis, or partial loss of motor power, (b) spasticity, or partial or total loss of voluntary motion accompanied by resistance to passive stretching, and (c) incoordination, namely motor power is present, but cannot be directed at its objective. These will now be considered separately.

PARALYSIS OR PARESIS

The typical picture of a stroke patient, that first comes to mind, is that of paralysis or paresis of one side of the body. This paralysis or paresis may, and often does involve the following: (a) the lower part of the face, the tongue and palate; (b) the upper extremity; (c) the trunk, and (d) the lower extremity. Each will be considered separately as each represents a different problem in stroke rehabilitation.

Facial Paralysis

The facial paralysis is of the so-called central type, as distinguished from the peripheral paralysis such as is seen in Bell's palsy. Since the upper part of the face is innervated from both sides of the brain, a cerebrovascular accident involving one hemisphere will spare the forehead and upper lid. The patient is able to wrinkle his forehead and open his eyes wide. However, the mouth is pulled to the nonparetic side by the nonparetic facial muscles, and the cheek will not be able to be retracted because of the weakness of the buccinator, and there will be a tendency of the cheek to balloon out. As a result, food particles will be retained on the paretic side, requiring mouth washing after meals, and sometimes cleansing of the cheek and gums by a sponge on a tongue depressor.

Paralysis of the Lips

If paralysis of the lips is severe, a mouth splint with rubber band (Fig. 8) around the ear will keep the lips from being pulled to the nonparetic side of the mouth. This can be worn constantly, or if the patient is embarrassed, it can be removed during the day and reapplied at night.

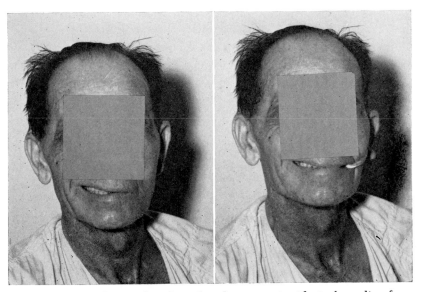

Figure 8. A simple mouth splint placed on paretic side to keep lips from being pulled to nonparetic side. a. *(left)* Mouth pulled to right. b. *(right)* Splint in place.

Paralysis of the Tongue

This type of paralysis can be detected by having the patient protrude his tongue, which will be seen to deviate to the paretic side by the push of the nonparetic muscles. This does not require any special treatment as it does not interfere with mastication. However, should the patient have a sharp or broken tooth, the tongue can be scratched; hence, the need for dental evaluation and treatment.

Nasopalatal Paralysis

Nasopalatal paralysis is occasionally seen as a stroke symptom. It is due to the involvement of the vertebrobasilar system and is usually associated with paresis of the intercostal muscles. It is manifested by weakness of phonation and shallow respiration. It represents a difficult treatment problem.

We had one such patient, a young man of twenty four, who suddenly developed a vertebral artery thrombosis, associated with a severe palatal paralysis and dysarthria. Stimulation of the palate with a sinusoidsal current resulted only in a mild improvement in phonation. An attempt to insert a palatal prosthesis by the dentist was not successful, as it caused the patient to gag. The only way the patient could communicate successfully without strain was by writing down his thoughts, and listening to the responses.

Trunk Muscle Paralysis

Paralysis of the trunk, including the abdominal muscles, is not at all uncommon in stroke patients. Examination of the abdomen will elicit a deviation of the linea alba and of the umbilicus to the nonparetic side. Weakness of the trunk muscles will tend to cause the patient to lean to the paretic side because the erector spinea is unable to keep the spine upright. This interferes with proper sitting, standing, walking, and will be considered later under ambulation.

Paralysis of Upper and Lower Extremities

The primary objective of stroke rehabilitation is to restore mobility to the patient. Ideally, this would be independent mobility without any assistive devices. This is not always possible, so we do the best we can in view of the degree of paralysis, from independent wheelchair ambulation to ambulation with cane and brace. Often we cannot accomplish even these, so we have to settle for dependent wheelchair ambulation or even permanent confinement to bed. The rehabilitation program which follows is geared to provide a progressive rehabilitation routine to take the patient to his maximum accomplishment. Before doing so, let us outline briefly the routine treatment of the upper and lower extremities, and the indications therefor.

Passive Exercise

The indication for passive exercise is that the patient is unable voluntarily to contract his limbs. Treatment consists of passive exercise by the therapist, by the therapist assistant, by a nurse or nurse assistant, by a member of the family, or by the patient himself using assistive devices or his nonparetic extremity. This should be done fifteen minutes, three times a day. (See Figs. 9-14 and Chapter 7, "Bed Exercise.")

Active Assistive Exercise

The indication is that the patient has weakness in his extremities, but some slight motion is possible, even if it is a trace. The treatment is active assistive exercise. The therapist or therapy assistant moves the joint through the range of motion and asks the patient to try and contract his muscles during such motion. (See Figs. 15-19.)

Active Exercise

Indication: The patient is able to move his joint through the range of motion without assistance. For treatment the patient is asked to perform active exercise. This means that he puts every functioning joint through the range of motion three times a day, at first under close supervision of the therapist and later on his own under general supervision. (See Fig. 20.)

Resistive Exercise

Indication: The patient's muscles have acquired enough

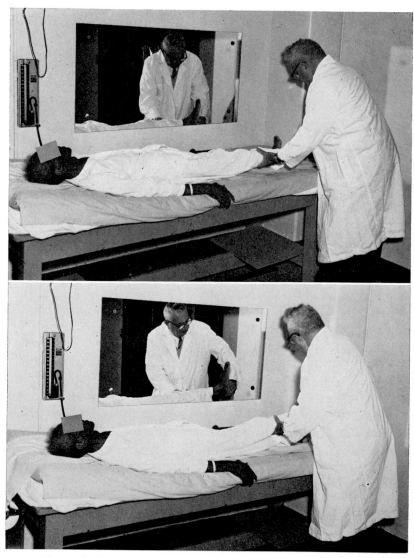

Figure 9. Passive exercise to right ankle. a. *(top)*, b. *(bottom)*.

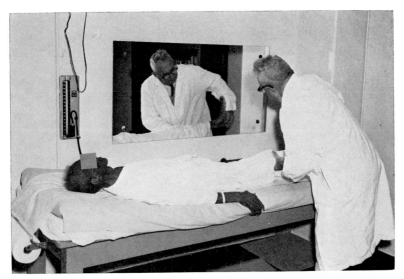

Figure 9c.

strength to be contracted against gravity. As treatment we then add resistive exercise. This would be particularly true of the non-paretic limbs, since so often they have to bear the burden of pre-hension and locomotion.

Rather than duplicate the exercise routine, we shall describe the exercises under discussion of the five phases of rehabilitation in the following chapter.

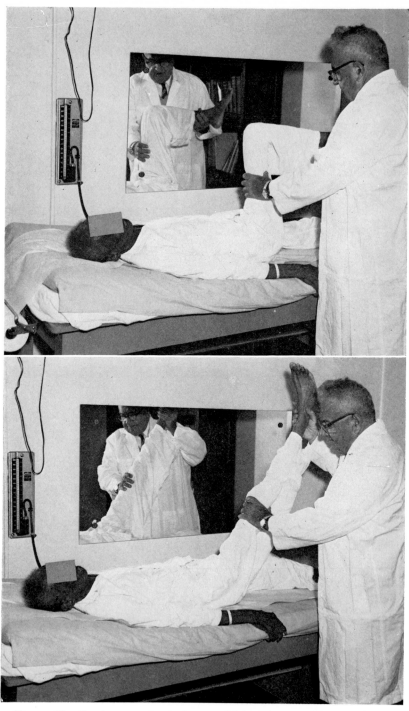

Figure 10a. Passive exercise to knee and hip. Flexion of knee and hip.

Figure 10b. Passive exercise—extension of knee, partial flexion of hip.

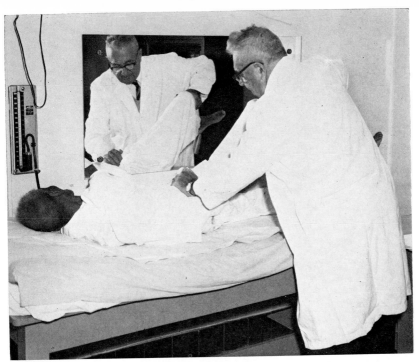

Figure 11. Abduction and internal rotation of hip.

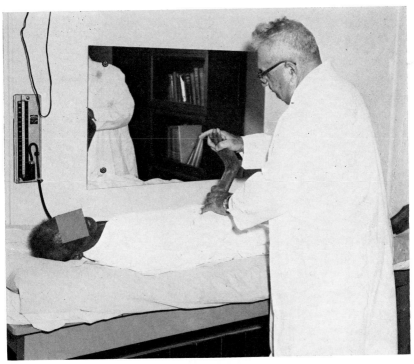

Figure 12. Dorsiflexion of wrist and fingers.

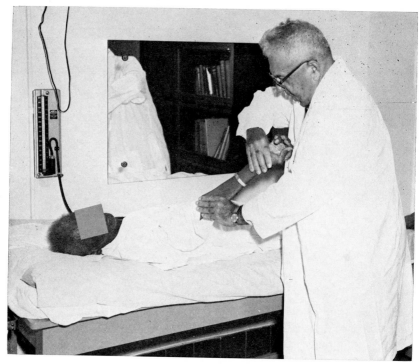

Figure 13. Pronation and supination of forearm.

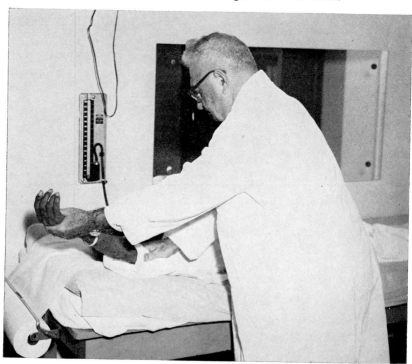

Figure 14. Extension of elbow and elevation of shoulder.

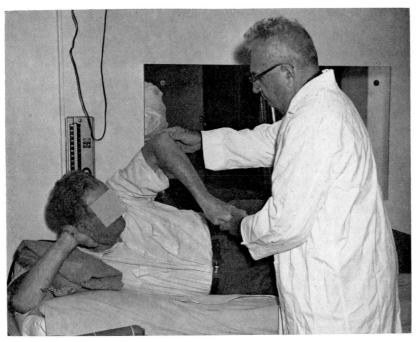

Figure 15. Figures 15 through 19 show active assistive exercise. The patient tries to move the part as the therapist takes the joint through range of motion. Figure 15a. *(top)*—Elbow extension; Figure 15b. *(bottom)*—Elbow flexion.

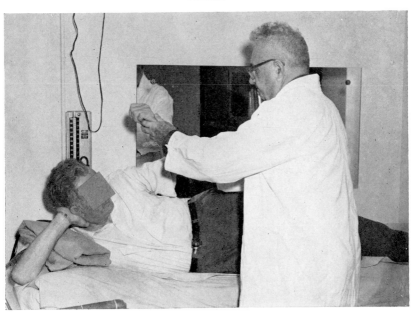

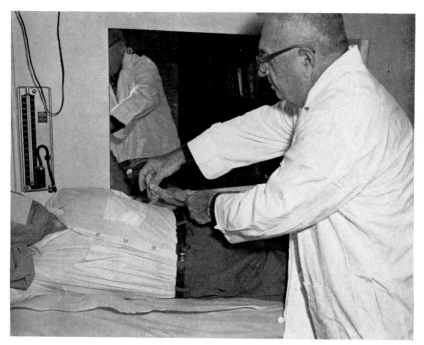

Figure 16. Active assistive exercise—thumb extension.

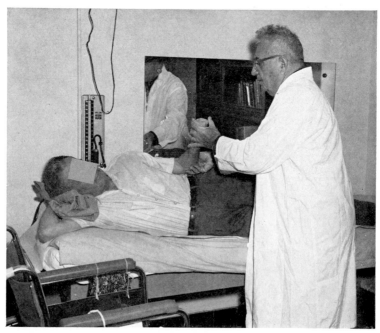

Figure 17. Active assistive exercise—forearm supination and pronation.

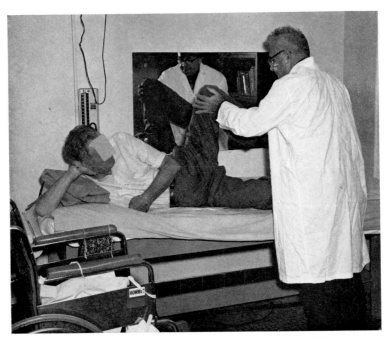

Figure 18. Active assistive exercise—knee extension and flexion.

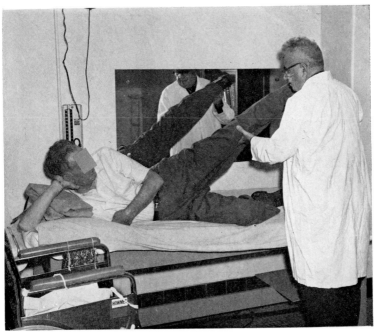

Figure 19. Active assistive exercise—hip abduction.

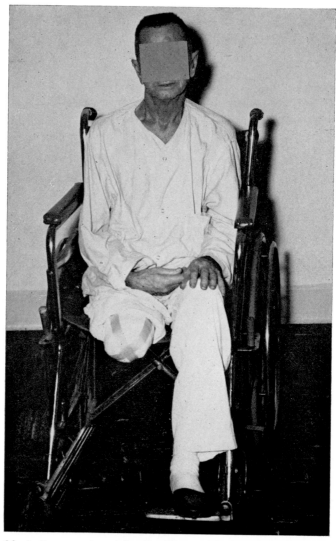

Figure 20. Active exercise—right shoulder, a. *(this page)* Shoulder adducted.

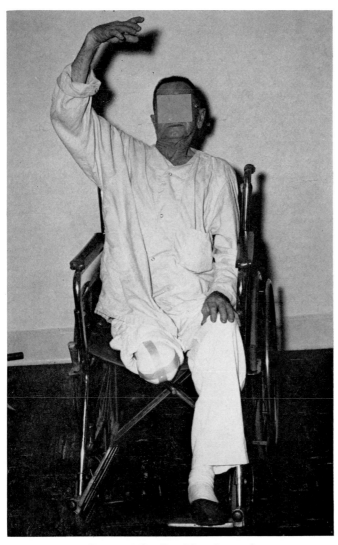

Figure 20b. Shoulder elevated.

Chapter 7

PROGRESSIVE REHABILITATION—THE BED PHASE (PHASE 1)

W HILE the restoration of function of the upper and lower extremities is the primary objective in the rehabilitation of a stroke patient, it cannot and should not be considered independently of the other problems of stroke management, namely bowel and bladder care and management of dysphasia and dysmentia. In this and in the following four chapters, however, we shall discuss mainly the physical rehabilitation program for a stroke patient under five phases: the bed phase, the wheelchair-dependent phase, the wheelchair-independent phase, the ambulatory-dependent phase, and finally, the ambulatory-independent phase.

The objects of the bed phase (phase 1) are to maintain the range of motion; to prevent contractures; to maintain and improve strength in the nonparetic upper and lower extremities; and to prevent the hazards of prolonged bed rest. Since this bed phase may last for more than a few weeks, it is advisable in the beginning to discuss the deleterious effects of bed rest.

BED REST—INTRODUCTION

A brief rest in bed after a stroke is not only desirable, but essential. Depending on the cause of the stroke and the patient's general condition, bed rest will be prescribed by the physician in charge for one or two days or for several weeks. A stroke due to embolism or thrombosis in a patient who has *no* associated systemic problems, such as fever, for example, will require only one or two days bed rest, while one due to hemorrhage will require a bed rest of three weeks or longer. Where the stroke is associated with coronary insufficiency or where the patient's vital signs are affected or where the patient is comatose or semicomatose, then bed rest will have to be prolonged beyond the three weeks, sometimes to a period of months. However, if such is the case, then in addition to the effects of the stroke itself, other deleterious changes begin to develop. Let us review some of these deleterious effects of bed rest.

PROLONGED BED REST—DELETERIOUS EFFECTS

Weldon[27] found that in four normal healthy young men, immobilization for six to seven weeks produced the following results: (a) an increase in nitrogen excretion, which in six to seven weeks amounted to the loss of four pounds of muscle protoplasm; (b) an increase in phosphorus, potassium, and sulfur excretion; (c) a fall in creatine tolerance, resulting from the inability of the muscle to store creatine and associated with a significant decrease in muscle mass and muscle strength; (d) an increase in urinary and fecal calcium; (e) an increase in urinary phosphorus, and in urinary pH, and a failure of urinary citric acid to parallel the rise in calcium, which is required for the formation of soluble calcium citrate, and as a consequence, the tendency for precipitation of calcium phosphate and formation of stones in the urinary tract; (f) a disturbance in homeostasis, with tendency to faint on assuming the erect position; (g) a decline of 5 percent in blood volume; and (h) a reduction in basal metabolic rate.

Further deleterious effects of bed rest, according to Dock,[28] are venous thrombosis, hypostatic pneumonia, constipation, fecal impaction, bone atrophy, edema of tissue, and danger of pulmonary edema. These results were confirmed by Ansel Keys.[29] And finally, as is well known, prolonged bed rest promotes muscle atrophy; the formation of pressure sores on the sacrum, trochanter, and malleoli; flexion contractures; and, as already indicated venous thrombosis and pulmonary embolism. To avoid these deleterious effects, it is necessary that a program of exercise be instituted early in all stroke patients, and this program should be maintained as long as the patient remains in bed and is inactive. This exercise program that we shall now describe is applicable to all stroke patients who are confined in bed.

The Bed

The bed should be a Hi-low® bed, so that it can be raised for the convenience of the personnel and lowered for the convenience of the patient. It should have provisions for elevating the head or legs. The mattress should be firm, not sagging, and for patients who will be confined long periods, it should be of the air or water type to prevent bed sores. At the head of the patient, a monkey bar should be installed so that the patient can help himself move from one place to another in bed by use of the nonparetic upper extremity. Side rails should be provided, so that the patient cannot fall out of bed. A cradle should be placed at the foot of the bed to keep the sheets off the patient's feet (Fig. 5-7).

Position of the Patient

The patient should be placed in the supine position, or on the nonparetic side. He should not be put on the paretic side for more than a few minutes for fear of developing pressure sores. He should not be put in the prone position, so as not to interfere with breathing. These latter positions may, of course, be used temporarily for the purpose of bed hygiene, but not for more than a short period of time required to minister to the patient. Early in the bed phase, the patient's paretic arm should be abducted, either by placing a pillow between the arm and chest, or by raising it in the Statue of Liberty position, alternating with the former. The postural alignment should be proper, as regards the head, neck, trunk, and lower extremities, and the fetal position, which the patient tends to assume, should be corrected. A sand bag at the outer side of the paralyzed foot will tend to prevent eversion; a foot-drop board at the sole of the foot will tend to overcome the danger of foot drop. A pillow between the thighs will obviate the tendency to adductor contracture. The patient should lie in bed with the paralyzed side nearest to the professional staff, that is if the bed is against the wall. Preferably, the bed should be so placed that the patient can be approached from all sides.

Bed Exercises

While the patient is in bed, he should be given passive exercise to the paretic limbs, and to the nonparetic limbs, unless he can cooperate by exercising the latter actively. The passive exercise should be done systematically, fifteen or more minutes three times a day, each joint being taken through its range of motion, five times at each session. The exercises should be given slowly, by the therapist, if available, by the nurse, if time permits, or by the rehabilitation therapy assistant, be he or she a physical therapy assistant or a nursing assistant. The exercises are as follows: (Remember you stand at bedside near the paralyzed part of the patient. See Figs 9 to 14.)

The Ankle

1. Place the contralateral hand (the one opposite the patient's paralyzed limb) under the patient's Achilles tendon, not under the knee or calf. You may do this by putting your hand any way which is most convenient for you, that is with your hand either on top of the leg and fingers underneath, or the hand and fingers underneath. This stabilizes the leg.
2. Place the homolateral hand (the one that corresponds to the paralyzed limb) under the heel of the patient.
3. Place your forearm under the sole of the patient's foot.
4. Slowly dorsiflex the ankle by pushing with your forearm against the sole of the foot, until the ankle is at 70 to 80 degrees to the horizontal. Hold it there for the count of seven, then release, rest and repeat.

The Knee and Hip

These are exercised together.
1. Place your homolateral hand under the patient's heel, and forearm under sole of foot, as in the ankle exercise.
2. Place your contralateral hand at the side of the patient's knee.
3. Flex the knee and hip, hold to the count of seven.
4. Extend the knee to 180 degrees, also to the count of seven.
5. Return to original position.

The Hand

1. Grasp the wrist with the contralateral hand.
2. Place your homolateral hand under the palm of the patient.

3. Dorsiflex the wrist to 45 degrees.
4. Slide your hand under fingers and dorsiflex the fingers to 0 position. (180° angle)
5. Hold to count of seven.
6. Return to original position and repeat.
7. Between treatments apply a wrist extension splint to wrist and fingers.

Elbow and Forearm

1. Place the contralateral hand under the elbow.
2. Place the homolateral hand around the wrist.
3. Extend and flex the elbow, and supinate the forearm—hold for count of seven.
4. Return to original position and rest and repeat.

Shoulder

1. Place your contralateral hand under the elbow.
2. Place the homolateral hand under the wrist.
3. Raise the arm forward in flexion to 180 degrees, hold seven seconds.
4. Abduct the shoulder so the arm is at 90 degrees to the body. Supinate forearm and keep forearm in supination seven seconds.
5. Return to original position.

Remember between treatments to keep pillows between shoulder and body, alternating with the Statue of Liberty position.

The Bladder

The bladder should be emptied at regular intervals by physician, nurse, or qualified aid, by catheterization, taking necessary aseptic precautions. We do not believe in inserting a permanent Foley catheter unless patient is unconscious more than forty-eight hours. The danger of infection is much greater from continuous catheterization than from intermittent catheterization. But, if sufficient help is not available, and a permanent Foley catheter is inserted, it should be opened at regular intervals, and the bladder should be irrigated with an antiseptc solution, as already mentioned under "Early Care"—Chapter 5, to prevent infection.

The Bowels

The bowels should be emptied by an enema until return is clear. Repeat every forty-eight hours.

Return of Consciousness

This program is continued as long as the patient is unconscious or semiconscious. On return of patient's consciousness, which will come within a variable period, depending on the cause and degree of the stroke, the rehabilitation team will orient the patient and his family on his condition and assume a more optimistic attitude.

For those muscles which are still completely paretic, passive exercise is continued as previously outlined. Where some muscular function has returned, active assistive exercise is instituted, as seen in Figures 15 through 19.

For the nonparetic muscles and for those paretic muscles in which this is possible, active exercises are recommended. (See Figure 20 a, b). The patient is also encouraged to use the nonparetic extremity with which to exercise the paretic limb. Figure 21 a, b shows a patient exercising his paretic right upper extremity by means of his functional left upper extremity. Should the patient not be able to hold the pulley strap, he is provided with a glove which is enclosed around the strap.

Patient Orientation

Assure the patient that if he cooperates, the chances are good for a satisfactory rehabilitation result. This is done even if the patient is aphasic and not responsive to directions, on the assumption that he understands what is said.

Reassure the family that prognosis, now that he has regained consciousness, is much better, that the patient has not lost his mind, even if aphasic, and that their attitude is very important to the patient and to the rest of the rehabilitation team. An attitude of hopefulness will tend to create a similar attitude in the patient and an attitude of helplessness, or negativism, will have a corresponding effect on the patient. The patient must be made to feel that he is wanted, no matter what, and he will make a better effort toward his recovery.

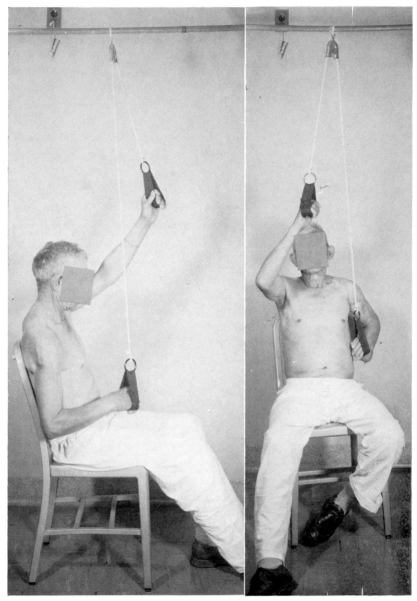

Figure 21. a. *(left)*, b. *(right)*. Exercise of the paretic right upper extremity by means of the nonparetic functional left upper extremity.

Bracing and Splinting

To prevent flexion contracture of the paretic wrist and fingers, we provide a wrist and finger extension splint. These splints can be made by the occupational therapy department. They usually are molded out of plastic materials and fitted to the wrist and fingers, either on the volar or dorsal aspect. There has been a great deal of discussion as to whether these splints should be placed anteriorly or posteriorly, the claim being that by applying an anterior splint, we stimulate the spastic muscles and encourage the development of flexion contractures. I have not found this to be so and prescribe either a volar or dorsal splint, whichever is more convenient for the patient. Recently, new plastic splint materials have been put on the market, permitting easy molding of the splint to the wrist and fingers by placing the material in hot water for a few minutes, thus allowing it to be shaped to the part. Five such materials are Bioplastic Tropical splints (Bioplastic Company), Prenyl (Ortho), Orthoplast (Johnson and Johnson), Royalite (Uniroyal), and Kydex (Rohm and Haas). Whatever splint is used, it is important to pad it with foam rubber to prevent skin irritation.

For the lower extremity, a short-legged foot-drop brace is often required to permit the patient to walk without dragging his toes or inverting his foot. Occasionally a long brace is needed to permit the patient to walk when the lower extremity remains flaccid, or to overcome a genu recurvatum, or to support a weak quadriceps. A knee cage is often adequate for this purpose (Fig. 22 a, b). An additional purpose of bracing of stroke patients, according to Perry,[30] is to produce position sense by substituting cutaneous touch and pressure for the lost proprioception in the tendons, joints, and muscles. The hospital brace shop, if available, can provide such a brace, or it can be purchased from any brace shop or surgical supply house.

The usual lower leg brace is fitted with a conventional or one-buckle T strap. Occasionally this type of strap exerts too much pressure on the medial malleous, thus encouraging the development of a pressure sore. To prevent such complications, Sam-

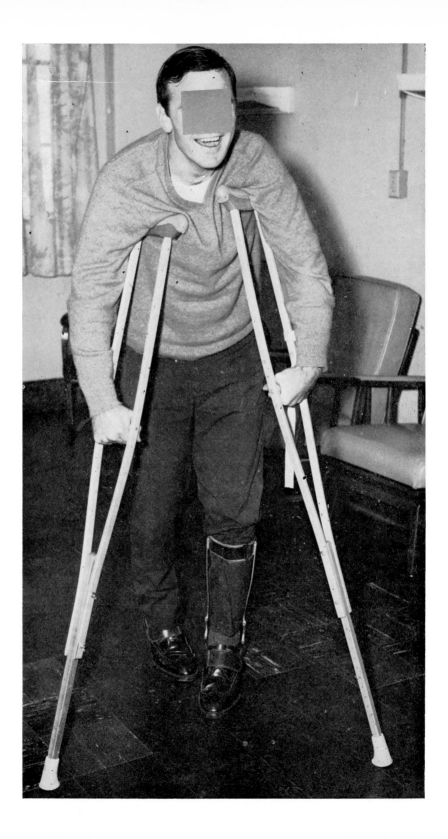

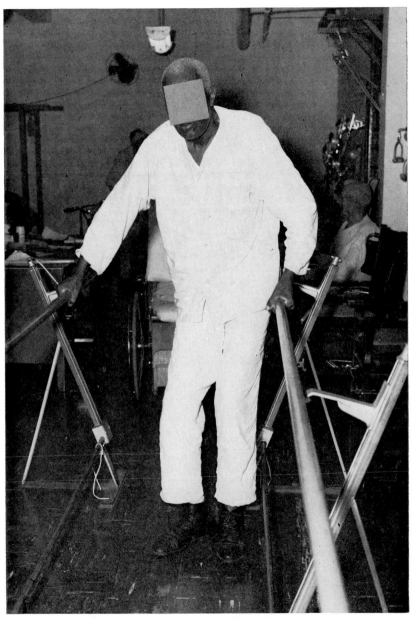

Figure 23. Stroke patient with weak right quad. a. *(this page)* Before.

Figure 22. Left foot-drop brace (Klenzak), for a patient with marked spasticity of plantar flexors. Note Velcro straps on both shoes.

«

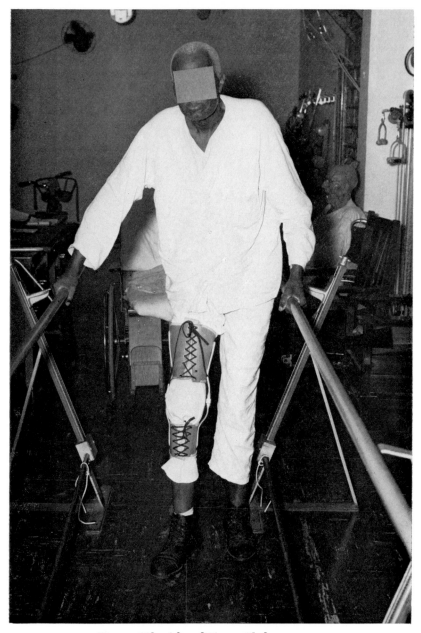

Figure 23b. After fitting with knee cage.

berg,[31] has proposed the fabrication of a two-buckle T strap which avoids this pressure.

Whenever we order a foot-drop brace, it has now become standard procedure to sew Velcro straps on *both* shoes so that the patient does not have to struggle with shoe tying. Where a T strap is prescribed, the usual buckle can also be replaced by a Velcro strap, which is much easier to fasten. Although Klenzak adjustable spring-type brace is not usually advisable for a foot-drop characterized by marked plantar spasticity, or severe ankle clonus, it is often the brace of choice, as its spring is adjustable and even removable, and thus it is quite comfortable. Where the Klenzak brace is not suitable, the usual order is for a short-legged brace with double bars, 90-degree stop, and a posterior metal calf band, with Velcro strap fastener stirrup attachment as above described. A good shoe, not necessarily orthopedic, is required (Fig. 23).

Chapter 8

WHEELCHAIR DEPENDENT PHASE (PHASE 2)

A T A variable time from the onset of the stroke, the patient's condition warrants his transfer from bed to wheelchair. Frequently this second phase is passed, and the patient enters immediately onto phase 3, namely wheelchair independence. Often, too, he skips phases 2, 3, and 4, and enters phase 5, namely ambulation independence. But let us assume that the patient follows the five-phase pattern, and the doctor authorizes his leaving the bed for wheelchair, but he has to be helped into and out of the wheelchair. He is also not able to propel his own wheelchair. Someone has to escort him. This is what we mean by wheelchair dependency. We shall discuss this phase from the standpoint of the wheelchair, transfer to, and from, and positioning.

THE WHEELCHAIR

The best wheelchair for stroke patients is a standard metal chair, with large wheels behind, and small wheels in front, with detachable arms, detachable and adjustable foot rests, removable head rest, and heel and toe loops to prevent foot from sliding off foot rest, and brakes. The wheelchair should be collapsible, so that it can be easily transported. It should be padded. One suggested pad is shown in Figure 24.

Wheelchair Transfer

This involves a transfer from the bed to the wheelchair and back to the bed. It is indicated when the patient does not have sufficient strength to transfer from the bed to the wheelchair and needs to be assisted.

1. Place the wheelchair at the side of the bed and lock the

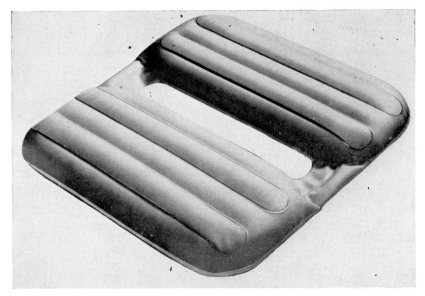

Figure 24. Pad for wheelchair.

brakes. Keep the chair on the nonparetic side of the patient.
2. Help the patient sit up in bed.
3. Turn the patient so that his feet hang over the edge of the bed.
4. Grasp the patient with both hands, one over each ilium.
5. Stand the patient in front of the bed; place both of your knees against the patient's knees to keep them from buckling.
6. Encourage the patient to grasp the far end of the wheelchair with non-paretic hand, but do not depend on this.
7. Assist the patient into wheelchair.

Wheelchair to Bed

See Figure 25 a-g.
1. Place the wheelchair at the side of the bed, so that the non-paretic side is nearest the bed.
2. Lock the brakes.
3. Grasp the patient with your hands over his iliac bones.
4. Place your knees against the patient's knees and help him stand, with most of his weight on his nonparetic leg.

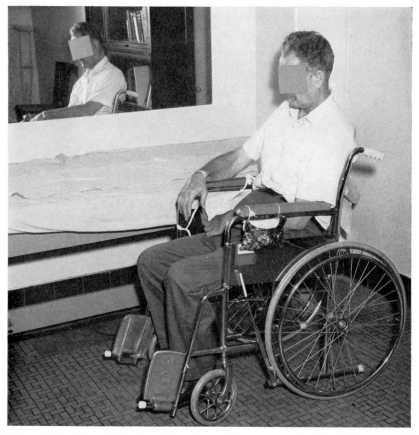

Figure 25a. Figure 25a through g shows the steps involved in *helping* weak patient go from wheelchair back to bed. a. *(this page)*.

5. Turn patient towards the bed; instruct him to place his non-paretic hand on mattress.
6. Help him sit on the mattress, gliding him back, so that both of his thighs are on mattress.
7. Lift his feet and turn them onto mattress, and help him lie down and assume correct posture.

The same procedure can be used to move the patient from the bed to the bedside commode. To escort the patient, be sure that his feet are placed in front of the heel loops and into the toe loops.

We have found that cushiony support at the paretic side of the

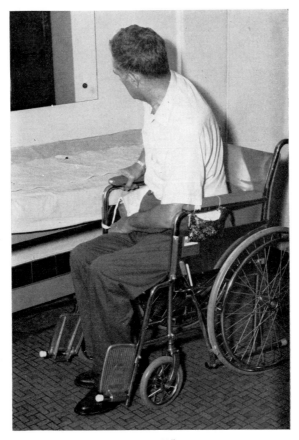

Figure 25b.

chair arms helps the patient to keep his arm supported with the
least discomfort (Figs. 54-57).

Bladder

As soon as the patient is able to stand up, the catheter, if it has
been inserted, is removed, and the patient is asked to void by
offering him a urinal, at the bedside if necessary, at regular intervals. If unsuccessful, and the patient cannot void and has to be
recatheterized, then another effort should be made in a few hours
for spontaneous voiding.

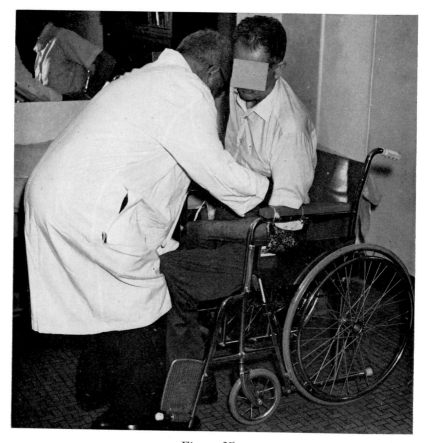

Figure 25c.

Bowels

When the patient is able to stand, he should be encouraged to move his bowels, at a bedside commode if necessary, or preferably, he should be assisted to the lavatory for this purpose. Here, it is important to know the patient's prestroke bowel habits and apply them. For example, if the patient has been in the habit of reading a newspaper or magazine while attempting the act of defecation, this procedure should be followed. If he required some prune juice, this should be given him. Laxatives should be avoided unless the patient has been accustomed to

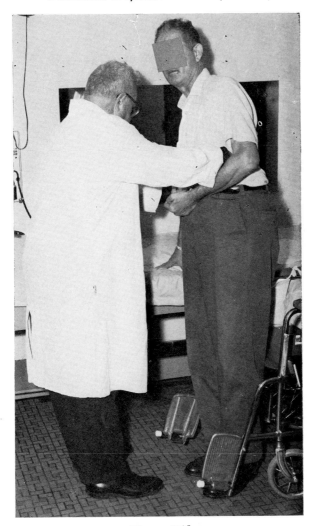

Figure 25d.

them, in which case a bowel-training program should be instituted as soon as feasible. This will be discussed in a later chapter (Chapter 21.)

Self-care

As soon as the patient has regained use of the nonparetic upper

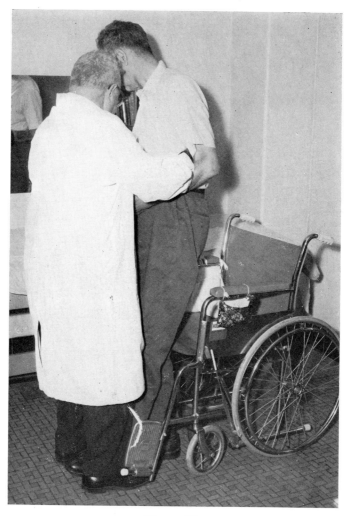

Figure 25e.

extremity, encourage him to undertake the simple self-care activities, such as feeding himself, shaving with an electric razor, combing his hair, brushing his teeth, and moving about in bed using the nonparetic limbs to assist the paretic limbs. For patients whose paretic extremity remains functionless, one-handed activities are encouraged. At this time, if the patient is in a Hi-low

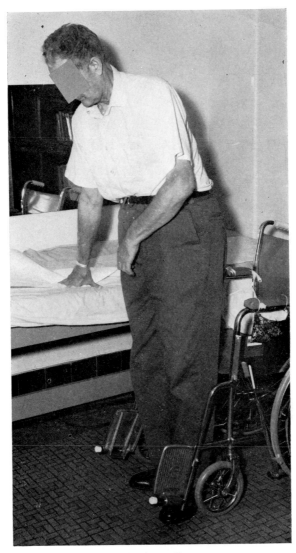

Figure 25f.

bed, it should be lowered. Otherwise, the patient should be moved to a low bed for easier transfer from bed to chair and vice versa.

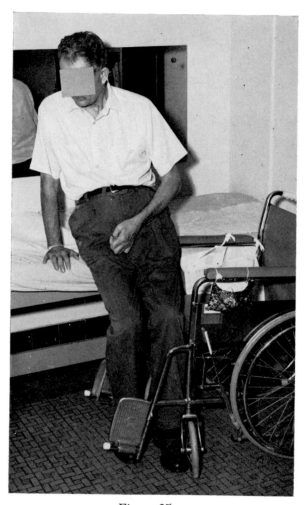

Figure 25g.

Chapter 9

WHEELCHAIR INDEPENDENT PHASE (PHASE 3)

Most patients following a stroke will be able to advance at least to this phase of wheelchair independence. Namely, they have the ability to get into and out of the wheelchair, to propel their wheelchair, and to take care of their daily needs.

In order for a patient to attain this objective, he has to meet the following requirements.

1. He has to be able to sit up without getting dizzy or blacking out.
2. He has to have at least one functioning upper extremity.
3. He has to have one functioning quadriceps femoris.

Given those three prerequisites, the patient may be expected with some training to become wheelchair independent.

FROM BED TO WHEELCHAIR

See Figure 26 a-f.

1. Place the chair near the bed.
2. Instruct the patient to place his nonparetic foot under his paretic ankle.
3. Have the patient press down on the mattress with his nonparetic hand.
4. Let his feet hang over the side of the bed for a minute or until he becomes adjusted to the vertical position. Ask him how he feels. If he feels dizzy, have him lie down again, and repeat later.
5. Bring the chair close to the patient, parallel with the bed, as in Figure 26 d.
6. Lock the brakes; make sure they are locked.
7. Ask the patient to stand on his nonparetic foot and grasp the distal hand rail of the chair with his nonparetic hand.

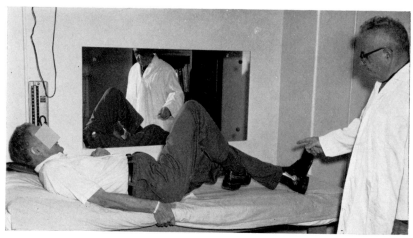

Figure 26. Figure 26 a. through f. shows the therapist *instructing* patient to
go from bed to wheelchair. a. *(top)*, b. *(bottom)*.

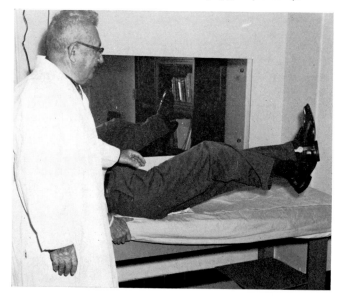

8. Rotating his body, the patient will then twist into the wheelchair and bring his paretic leg next to his nonparetic leg.

9. He will complete the procedure by adjusting himself to the
wheelchair with whatever power he has in his nonparetic
hand.

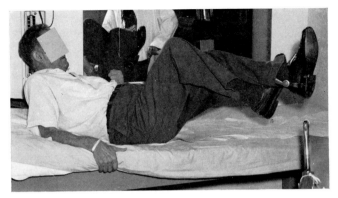

Figure 26c. *(top)*, d. *(bottom)*.

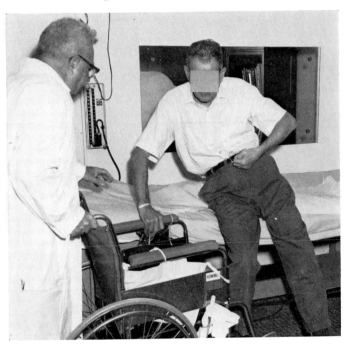

10. With his nonparetic hand he will place his paretic foot into the foot pedal loops so that it is prevented from falling off.

11. Teach the patient to release the brakes, and then he is ready for wheelchair ambulation.

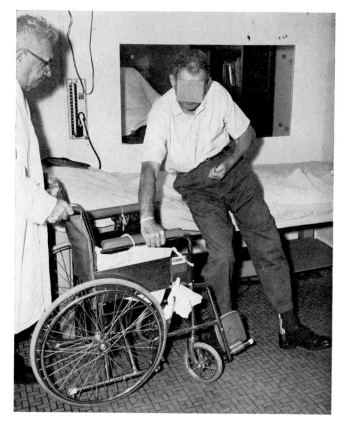

Figure 26e.

Wheelchair Ambulation (Propulsion)

The patient propels his wheelchair either forward or backward.

Forward Propulsion

1. Check the brakes; be sure they are released.
2. Put both feet on the pedals.
3. With the nonparetic hand rotate forward, alternately, the right or left rear wheel, followed by rotating the opposite wheel.
4. If the patient's hand is not strong enough to rotate the wheel, he may need an assist, namely, extension bars at-

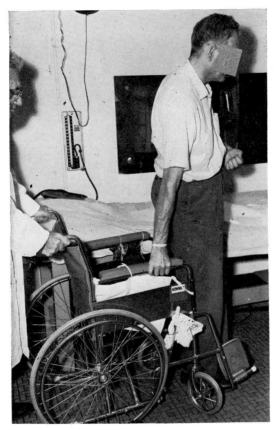

Figure 26f.

tached to the top of outer wheels. These bars can be either horizontal or vertical, the former for grasping, the latter for propelling.

Alternate Forward Propulsion (Fig. 27)
1. Same as above.
2. Raise the pedal on the nonparetic side and push foot backward against the ground as the wheels go forward.

Backward Propulsion
Some patients prefer to manipulate the wheels by backward propulsion.

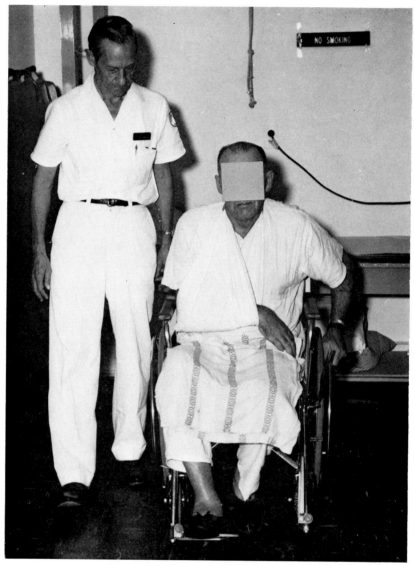

Figure 27. Patient being instructed in forward wheelchair propulsion.

1. Again, be sure the brakes are released.
2. Raise the foot pedal of the nonparetic leg.
3. Keep the foot and the toe of the paretic leg in the loops of the foot pedal.
4. Alternately push the rear wheels backward, and push forward against the ground with the nonparetic foot, so that the wheelchair moves backward.

The return to bed is similar to that in Chapter 8, except that the patient is now able to help himself better.

Chapter 10

AMBULATORY DEPENDENT PHASE (PHASE 4)

WITHIN a few days after the onset of the stroke, the flaccid, paralyzed lower extremity, usually, gradually becomes spastic. In only a few cases does the flaccidity remain permanent. These latter patients present a problem which will be discussed later. The majority of patients, however, do show an increasing spasticity of the lower as well as the upper extremity. While in the upper extremity this spasticity presents a problem which hinders rehabilitation, in the case of the lower extremity, the spasticity actually is an assistive device that helps with ambulation retraining. The reason is that in the case of the lower extremity the spasticity is of the extensor thrust type, characterized by a spastic gluteus maximus and medius, spastic quadriceps, and spastic plantar flexors. The former, i.e. the spastic hip and knee extensors, tend to support the body during standing and walking. The spastic plantar flexors, on the other hand, interfere with ambulation in that during the swing phase, the leg has to be elevated sufficiently high enough to lift the foot off of the floor.

The answer to ankle-plantar flexor spasticity, if mild, is a narrow lift on the opposite shoe which will permit the patient to walk with minimal difficulty. If the spasticity is severe and the ankle goes into marked plantar flexion during the swing phase, then a foot-drop brace will have to be provided for the patient, so as to permit his foot to clear the floor. (See Chapter 7, "Bracing and Splinting.") Because of the weakness of the hip and knee flexors, as the patient lifts his foot, he tends to hike his pelvis by using the trunk muscles rather than the hip and knee flexors, thus producing a circumduction gait so typical of these patients. In the younger individual, an attempt is made to overcome this gait

80

deviation by special training. But, in the older patient we do not make such effort, since it is wasteful of the therapist's time and unnecessary. What we are interested in is that the patient can walk, with a satisfactory gait, if possible, but if this is impossible or impractical, then with any gait, so long as he does walk.

The program for *ambulation training* of a patient with a spastic paralyzed lower extremity is carried out in four steps:

1. The patient is ordered active exercises to the nonparetic lower extremity starting with the patient in bed and continuing when he is able to get out of bed. At the same time, passive exercises are given to the paretic lower extremity to prevent contractures, to maintain range of motion, to promote the return of circulation, and to prevent atrophy from disuse. These exercises have already been illustrated. (See Chapter 7.)

2. When the patient's condition warrants, as determined by the physician in charge, he is assisted with standing at the bedside by a therapist or by nursing personnel. The object of this is (a) To help reestablish homeostatis, (b) To develop proprioception in the lower extremity, (c) To promote extensor thrust and encourage the lower extremity to assume the extended position. If the patient has been in bed for several days and he cannot stand without a feeling of faintness, then he is placed on a tilt table, and the table is gradually tilted to the vertical position until the patient can stand for a few minutes without blacking out.

3. When the patient is able to stand, on both feet with therapist assistance, then human assistance is replaced by mechanical assistance, i.e. a walker, or preferably, parallel bars. The patient is placed behind the walker, or behind the parallel bars and taught to stand first on his nonparetic lower extremity, and then to straighten his paretic lower extremity, until he can bear weight on it.

4. He grasps the walker or one of the parallel bars with his nonparetic hand and glides his paretic hand on the other bar. In the case of the walker, he holds on with both hands and propels first the nonparetic leg and then the paretic leg.

In the case of the parallel bars, he propels first the nonparetic leg and paretic hand, then the paretic leg and nonparetic hand, alternately. He does this until he has attained some confidence with his ambulation.

This phase is also for patients who have the strength to walk, provided that someone supervises their ambulation or actually helps to support them. These patients may use a crutch or cane, and brace, but still cannot be left to walk alone, because of weakness, incoordination, marked clonus, or disequilibrium. Patients with anosognosia should always be supervised during ambulation, because ignoring the involved leg, they will leave it far behind with each step, and in trying to catch up, may fall. More about anosognosia later.

ADDITIONAL INSTRUCTIONS
From Bed to Standing

Review Chapter 9.

1. Repeat as in Chapter 9, letting your feet hang over edge of bed.
2. Get hold of a cane or crutch with the nonparetic hand.
3. Get off the bed with the nonparetic leg, holding onto the cane with the nonparetic hand.
4. Bring the paretic leg and the paretic hand off bed.
5. Bring the cane forward, in the beginning, no more than six inches.
6. Bring the nonparetic leg forward next to the cane.
7. Bring the paretic leg forward next to the nonparetic leg.
8. Rest and repeat.

If the patient is very weak, an attendant will have to hold on to him either by the belt, or by the arm. If the patient is fairly strong and can walk alone, the attendant will stand close to the patient and be ready to catch him if he starts to fall. (Figs. 28 to 34 show the progressive stages of teaching a patient to walk with therapist's assistance or under his supervision, with a crutch or cane, up and down steps and ramp, Fig 34 a and b shows how we teach a patient the proper way to lift an object from the floor. "Bend your knees and hips, keep your head up.")

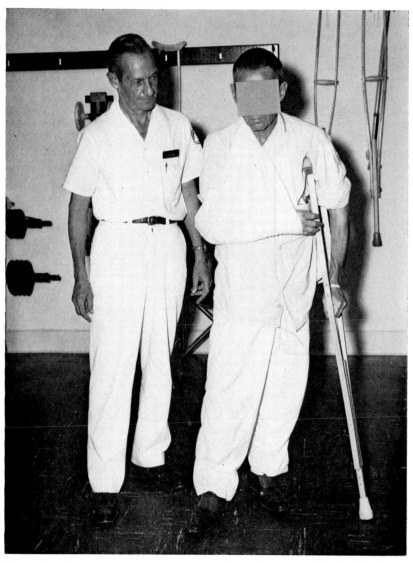

Figure 28. Figures 28-34—dependent ambulation, i.e. with therapist's assistance. Figures 28 and 29—ambulation with single crutch with therapist's assistance.

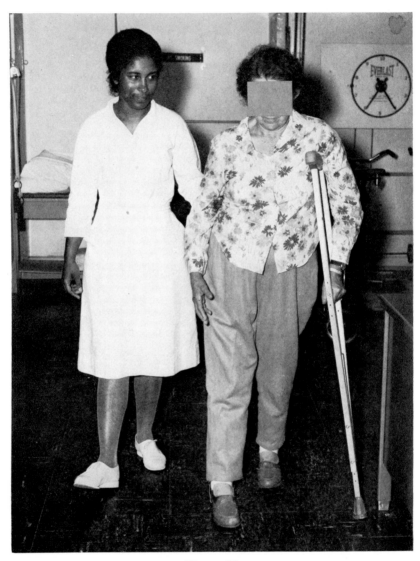

Figure 29.

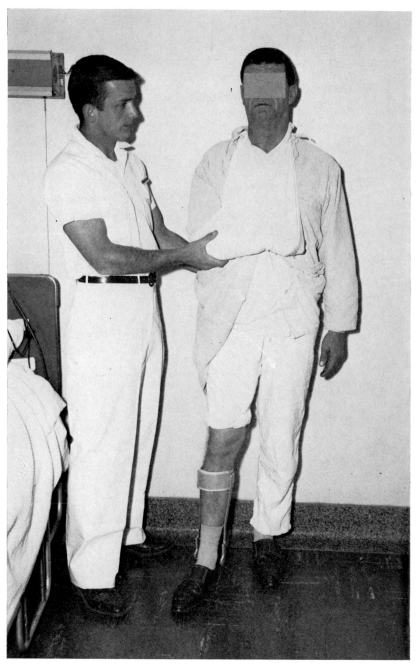

Figure 30. Figures 30 and 31—ambulation without support, but with therapist's assistance.

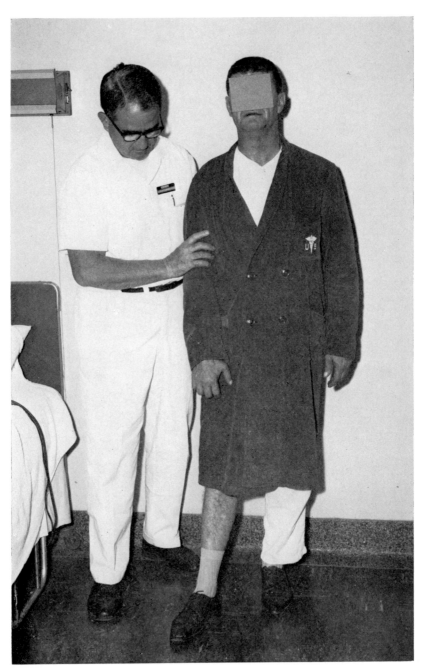

Figure. 31.

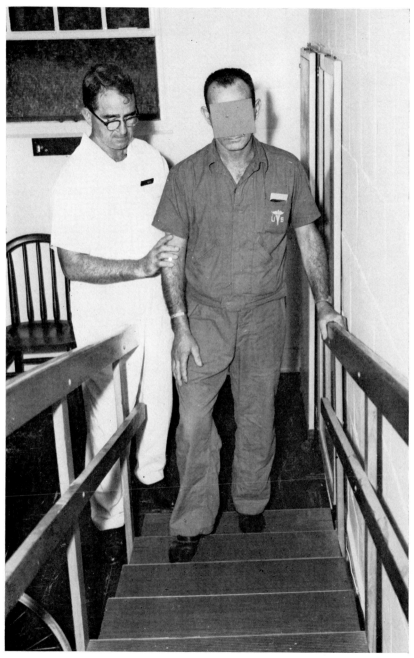

Figure 32. Instructing patient to go down steps, holding on to bannister with therapist's assistance.

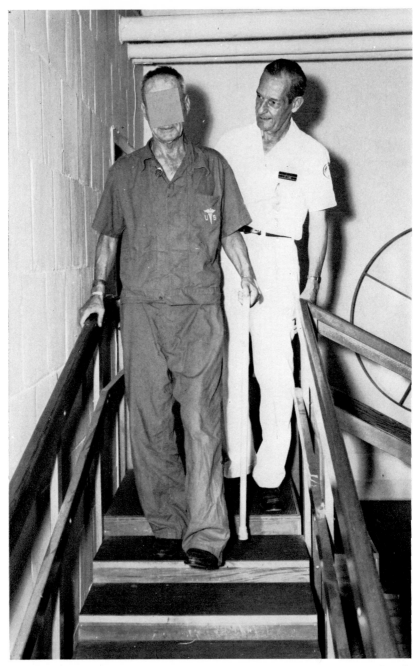

Figure 33. Instructing patient to go down steps, with cane in paretic hand, nonparetic hand holding on to bannister, therapist watching but not holding on to patient. Note: If patient's paretic hand can not hold cane, it can be placed between arm and chest.

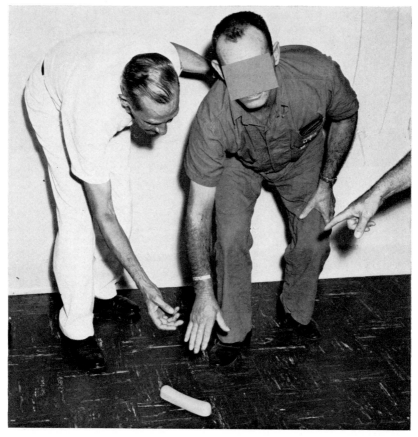

Figure 34 a. *(this page)* and b. show patient being taught proper way to lift an object from floor. "Bend at the knees and hips. Keep your head up." (Note: The corrective therapist, Mr. J. B. Cobb, one of the best, has since died.)

From Wheelchair to Walking

1. Always lock the brakes.
2. Bring the body forward to the edge of the chair.
3. Grasp the cane or crutch (which has been placed near the chair or which is being held by the attendant).
4. Put the weight on the cane and the nonparetic leg at the same time.

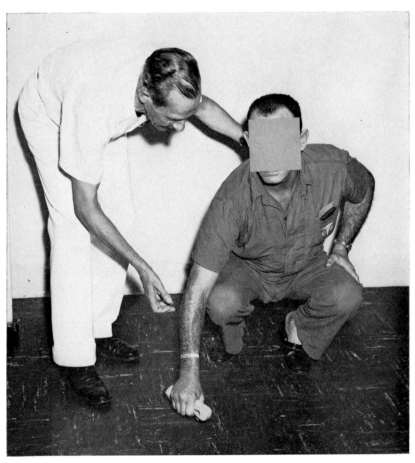

Figure 34b.

5. Stand, taking the paretic leg off wheelchair.
6. Repeat, as in preceding 5, 6, and 7.

Back to Bed from Walking

1. Step close to the bed.
2. Press down on the cane and the nonparetic leg, slide onto the mattress and put the cane to one side.
3. Slide back into bed.

Back to Wheelchair from Walking

1. Step close to the wheelchair.
2. Be sure the brakes are locked.
3. Bring the nonparetic foot to the side of the chair.
4. Grasp the arm of the chair with the nonparetic hand.
5. Slide into the chair, carrying the paretic thigh into it.

Chapter 11

INDEPENDENT AMBULATION PHASE (PHASE 5)

For patients whose paretic lower extremity is functional, independent ambulation is possible even if one upper extremity is completely useless (Figs. 35-40).

PROGRESSIVE ROUTINE

Wheelchair to Parallel Bars

1. Have the patient go from his bed to the wheelchair as in Chapter 9.
2. Have him wheel himself to the parallel bars.
3. Lock the brakes on the wheelchair.
4. Grasp one bar with the nonparetic hand.
5. Press down on the nonparetic hand and on the nonparetic leg.
6. Stand up between the parallel bars.
7. Advance the nonparetic hand on bar.
8. Move the nonparetic foot forward.
9. Bring the paretic functional leg to the side of nonparetic leg.
10. Glide the paretic hand on the bar up to the level with the nonparetic hand.
11. Repeat.

Back to Wheelchair

1. Stand on the nonparetic foot.
2. Turn on this foot and grasp the opposite bar with the nonparetic hand.
3. Slide or ease the paretic hand off bar and place it on the opposite bar.
4. Walk back to wheelchair, which faces the parallel bars.
5. Grasp the opposite side of the chair with the nonparetic hand.

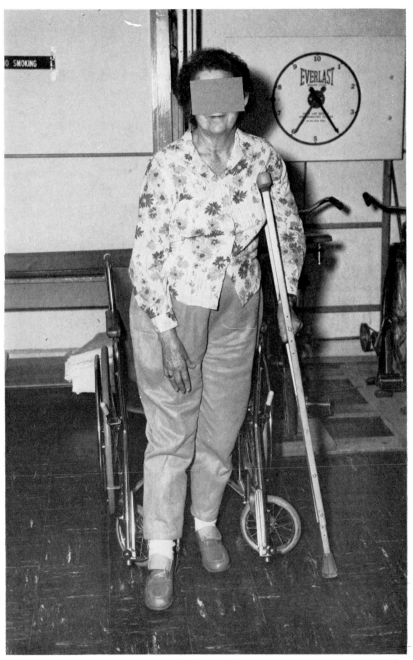

Figure 35. a. *(this page)* and b. show two views of patient walking with a single crutch and right foot-drop brace. Note Velcro straps on both shoes.

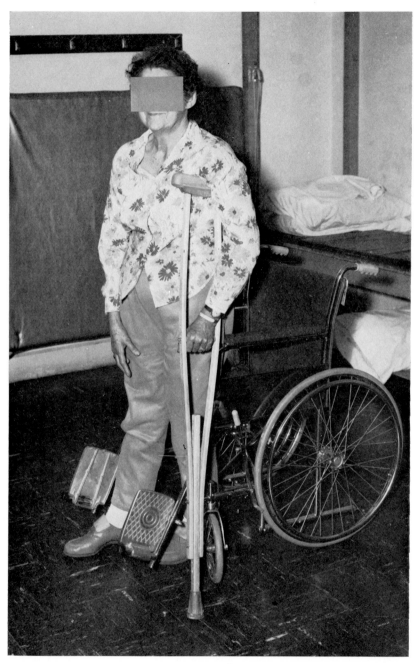

Figure 35b.

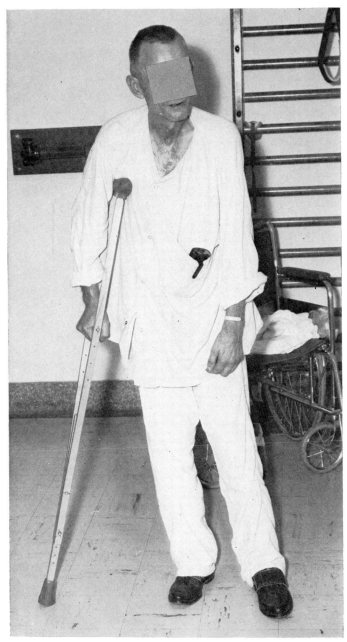

Figure 36. Patient walking with wood crutch.

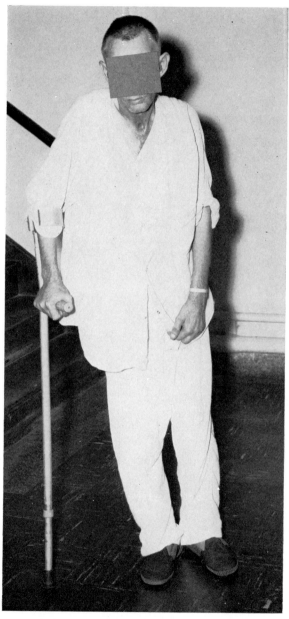

Figure 37. Same patient walking with aluminum crutch.

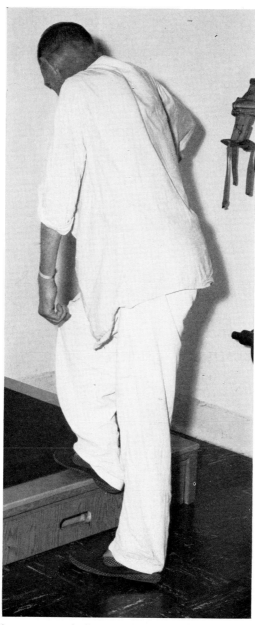

Figure 38. Patient being taught to walk up step (a., *this page*) with cane.

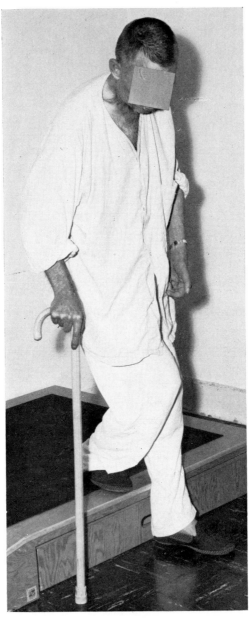

Figure 38b. Patient being taught to walk down step with cane.

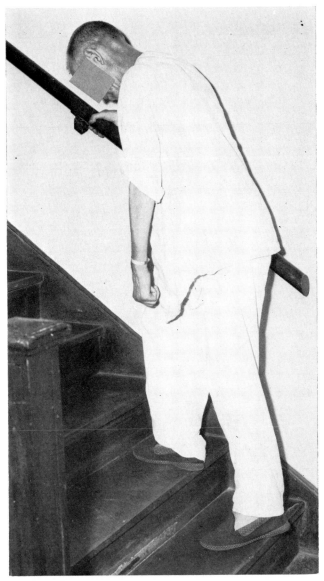

Figure 39. Patient being taught to walk up steps, holding on to bannister. (a., *this page*).

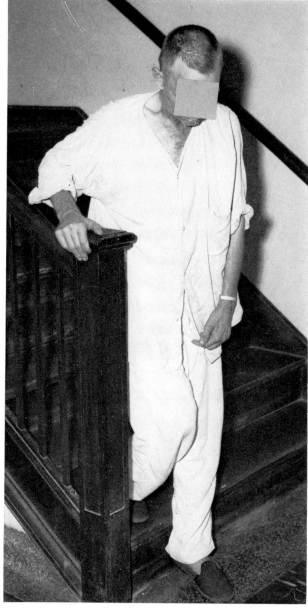

Figure 39b. Patient being taught to walk down steps, holding on the bannister.

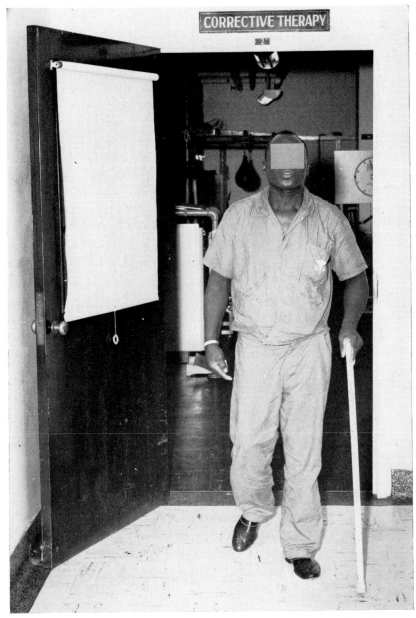

Figure 40. Patient walking with cane. Note—posture. Patient has been instructed to keep head and body slightly forward, to prevent falling backward.

6. Turn and place the buttocks into the wheelchair.
7. Slide the body into the chair.

Wheelchair to Cane

The patient is given a cane to hold in his nonparetic hand. The cane then acts as a partial replacement for the paretic upper extremity. He is asked to advance the nonparetic lower extremity, stabilizing the paretic limb and cane, then to advance simultaneously the paretic leg and cane, then again the nonparetic leg, etc. First he stays between the parallel bars, using them for psychological support. When he has reached a satisfactory stage in walking between parallel bars, he is allowed to leave the bars and walk outside them, at first with supervision, and when the therapist feels he is ready, he is allowed to walk independently. Once he has reached this stage, he has no problem going from bed to cane.

Steps and Ramp

The next step is to teach the patient to walk up and down steps, and up and down a ramp. To walk up the steps, the patient stands in front of the bottom step and faces it. He places the nonparetic foot on the first step, keeping the paretic foot on the ground. He next lifts the paretic foot and cane and places them on the step next to the nonparetic foot. If the patient has difficulty in negotiating the steps with his cane, he is asked to place the cane between the paretic arm and chest and to use his nonparetic hand to pull him up the steps. For greater safety, the patient should use the bannister.

Descending the Steps

Here the positions of the legs are reversed, namely the patient is taught to go down with his paretic foot first to be followed by the cane and his nonparetic foot.

Occasionally a patient prefers to go down the steps backwards. Here it is better for him to hold on to the bannister with the nonparetic hand, go down first with the paretic leg, to be followed by the nonparetic leg.

Ramp Ambulation Instructions

The instructions are the same as for step ambulation.

Independent Ambulation Outdoors

To make the patient completely independent, he should be taught to learn to walk outdoors, to negotiate crossing the street with the light, to go up and down the sidewalk and up and down building steps, to go through a turnstile, and to go in and out of elevators and up and down an escalator. He should also be taught how to pick up objects from the floor (Fig. 34 a, b), and how to get into and out of an automobile (Fig. 41 a, b).

Use of Cane or Crutch

For younger stroke recovered patients who have good coordination, consideration should be given to the discarding of a cane. But for the older hemiplegic disabled, it is best to provide them with a cane or even with a crutch. These patients should be taught to walk slowly and pause after each double step.[32] Often these patients will not be able to walk independently, and we must revert to dependent ambulation with constant supervision. Too many patients have fallen and broken their hips for us to permit the family or rehabilitation team to forget this rule. Before leaving this subject, it is advisable to mention some *contraindications to independent ambulation*. These are the following:

1. Cardiac decompensation.
2. Mental deterioration.
3. Severe spasticity, manifested by marked clonus. It is always best to have someone walk beside the patient.
4. Incoordination.

Finally, here are a few simple rules:

1. Try to have the patient walk a few minutes every hour, all day.
2. Provide the patient with a short leg brace, if there is a permanent foot drop. Not only will it permit the patient to walk better, but what is just as important, a short leg brace saves 40 percent energy.[33]

And here is a final word of caution: Remember that the patient tends to lean to the paretic side, thus facing the danger of falling. Remind him to lean slightly to the nonparetic side and forward thus reducing the tendency to fall. Throughout all these ambulation training sessions the patient is reminded constantly to exer-

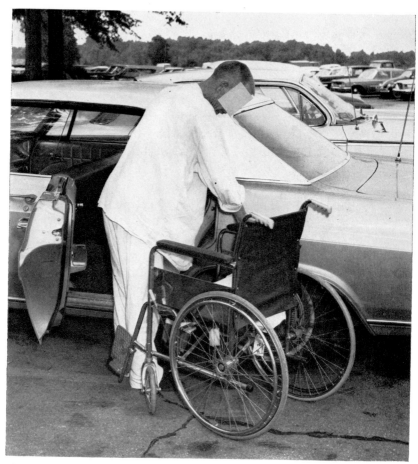

Figure 41. Patient being instructed to get into automobile (a., *this page*).

cise his paretic upper extremity using the nonparetic extremity as an assist (Fig. 42).

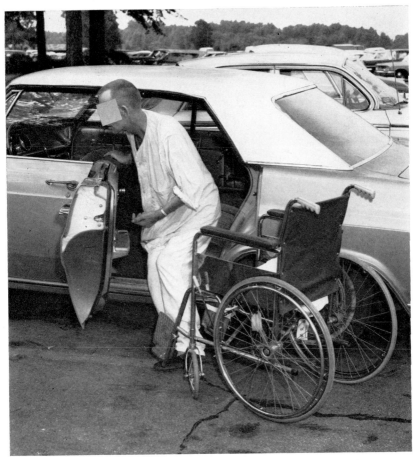

Figure 41b. Patient being instructed to get out of automobile.

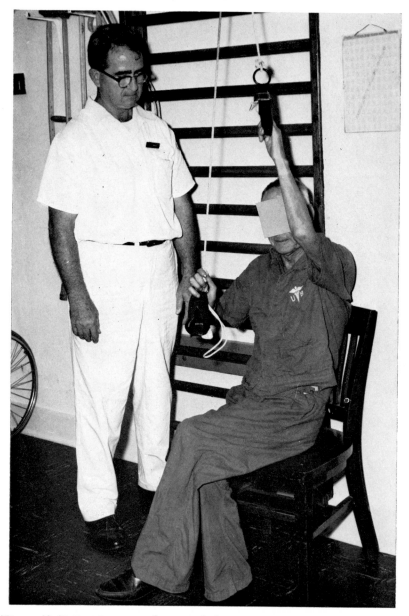

Figure 42. Patient is constantly reminded to exercise paretic upper extremity with the help of nonparetic extremity.

Chapter 12

S.A.E. (STIMULATION ASSISTIVE EXERCISE)

HISTORY

IN 1956, when I was appointed Chief, Physical Medicine Rehabilitation, Veterans Administration Hospital, Durham, North Carolina and Associate in Rehabilitation, Duke University School of Medicine, I undertook a clinical research project to see if we could improve function in the paralyzed upper extremity of stroke patients. The idea was to use electrical stimulation applied to paralyzed muscles while the patient was asked to attempt to contract these muscles. In other words, the object was to replace the therapist's assistive part of active assistive exercise with stimulation, hence the name Stimulation Assistive Exercise, or S.A.E.

I was fortunate in obtaining funds for a research assistant, a full-time physical therapist. The S.A.E. routine was instituted in 1956, and the results were reported in 1960.[39] Out of a total of twenty-seven patients treated, ten (37%) had excellent recovery of function; ten (37%) had a satisfactory recovery, and seven (26%) showed no improvement. The treatment and its results were publicized by the Veterans Administration central office and by the administrator of the Veterans Administration. Then came the deluge, inquiries from all over the United States and from many foreign countries, from professional and from lay people who were looking for a panacea for stroke paralysis, and who were given the impression that S.A.E. was such a panacea.

The following paragraphs will indicate that it is no panacea and will, I hope, put S.A.E. in its proper perspective.

INTRODUCTION

Immediately following a stroke, while the medical team is

attempting to pinpoint the diagnosis and save the life, the object of the rehabilitation team is to maintain range of motion, to promote circulation, and to prevent contractures.

Since the paralyzed upper extremity is flaccid, all of these objectives can be attained by passive exercise (Chapters 5 and 7, Figs. 9 through 14). This is accomplished by having the physical therapist and the ward personnel take each joint slowly through a complete range of motion. The shoulder is passively flexed, extended, externally and internally rotated, abducted, and adducted and elevated; the elbow is flexed, extended; the thumb is opposed to the little finger. This passive exercise is continued by the members of the rehabilitation team at least three times a day, as long as the limb remains flaccid. When spasticity sets in, the range of motion exercise is continued until either there is some sign of return of voluntary motion or until the team is convinced that further recovery is improbable. The cut-off time is generally considered to be two months. If, in two months, there is no return of function, then no return should be expected, and one may proceed on the assumption that the arm will remain paralyzed. If, at some future time, spasticity sets in, then reevaluation is called for and perhaps a new effort at retraining.

In most cases, however, within a few days, the flaccid arm does gradually become spastic, and the members of the rehabilitation team continue to carry out passive exercise. Then, following a variable interval, one will notice the development of some voluntary motion, usually in the shoulder abductors, although any part of the extremity may be the first to exhibit active motion.

Further management will then depend upon the attitude of the rehabilitation team. In some centers, an attempt is made to improve function by active assistive exercise (Figs. 15-19), but often there is only a minimal degree of active motion, and in many cases, a helpless attitude will result. There is cessation of all further effort at attempting to improve function in the paralyzed upper extremity, and all emphasis is upon self-care and ambulation. This attitude which seems so prevalent is not justified. Numerous workers in the field of stroke rehabilitation have shown that proper exercise, by trained personnel, for an adequate time, will often result in an improvement in function of the spastic paralyzed upper extremity. Even if the arm does not become completely functional, but merely attains the status of an assistive limb, it would still be worthwhile to continue the effort. Some of these exercises will now be described.

METHODS OF NEUROMUSCULAR REEDUCATION

Kabat[34] has described a series of exercises aimed to induce the greatest possible activity in the paretic muscles with each voluntary effort in order to accelerate recovery. Since in stroke paralysis the involved cerebrospinal tract is permanently damaged, an effort is made to open new pathways in the central nervous system by strong excitation. With this aim in mind, Kabat induced maximal excitation by maximal resistance, reflexes, irradiation, and successive induction. Kabat has developed several tables indicating how to accomplish these irradiation patterns for different joint involvements.

Temple Fay,[35] used pathological reflexes, such as the Babinski or Marie-Foix, to promote return of function in an involved spastic extremity. He claimed that repeated exercise by a trained therapist would result in such improvement.

The Bobaths, on the other hand,[36] believe in inhibition rather than excitation of reflexes. While most of the work has been done with children, they feel that similar results can be obtained with the adult spastic hemiplegic. As an example, they stretch the flexors of the elbow where there is a spastic flexion contracture, for the purpose of relieving the spasticity.

Rood,[37] stimulates cutaneous and proprioceptive nerve endings to accomplish motion or relaxation.

Taking an entirely different approach, Psaki and Treanor,[38] emphasize control of afferent impulses in the management of spastic paralysis. They inhibit such afferent impulses by (a) restriction of standing and ambulation, (b) selective reeducation of extensors of upper extremity and flexors of the lower extremity, (c) curtailment of occupational therapy and activities of daily living, to gross movements, and (d) interruption of conduction of the afferent impulses by nerve blocks and even by surgery.

While these methods in skilled hands may produce satisfactory results, they have one common objection: They all require a great deal of time by highly skilled personnel. To obviate this objection, a method of neuromuscular reeducation has been developed by the author; it is called S.A.E. for stimulation assistive exercise.[39]

The prerequisites for the employment of S.A.E. are (a) the paralysis is spastic. (b) There is some recovery of function. (c) The patient has to be able to respond to simple instructions. The advantage of S.A.E. is that it can be administered even at home, by nonprofessional personnel.

The technique is as follows: The patient is seated near a plinth or table; a three-inch by three-inch electrode is attached to the abductors of the shoulder or extensors of the elbow and extensors of the wrist and fingers (Fig. 43 a, b). They are connected by cords to a sinusoidal machine that delivers six to ten stimuli per minute. The patient is instructed, when he feels the current, to

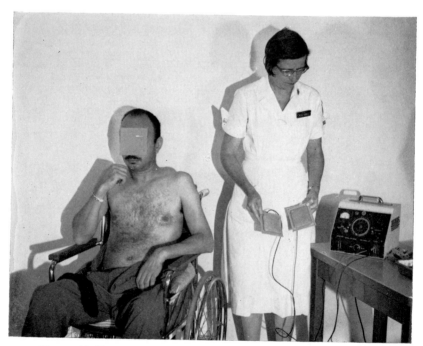

Figure 43. Equipment required for S.A.E. routine (a., *this page*).

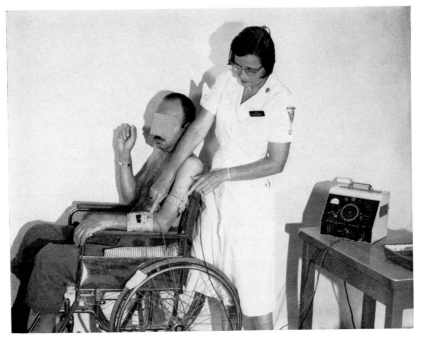

Figure 43b. Electrodes attached to patient's arm and forearm.

attempt to abduct the shoulder, extend the elbow, supinate the forearm, and extend the wrist and fingers. According to Sherrington's law of reciprocal innervation, when the agonists are stimulated, the antagonists relax (Fig. 44). Since in stroke paralysis the spasticity involves primarily the adductors of the shoulder, flexors or the elbow, pronators of the forearm, and flexors of the wrist and fingers, stimulation of the abductors of the shoulder or extensors of the elbow and extensors of the wrist and fingers will cause the spastic muscles to relax, offering the patient an opportunity to exercise the stimulated muscles. The S.A.E. is given thirty minutes, two times per day. Any sinusoidal machine will do, provided it delivers stimuli at the rate of six to ten per minute. A greater frequency does not give the stimulated muscles a chance to relax. Figure 45 a and b shows patient receiving S.A.E. treatment for a paretic right upper extremity.

It is necessary for someone interested in the patient to remind

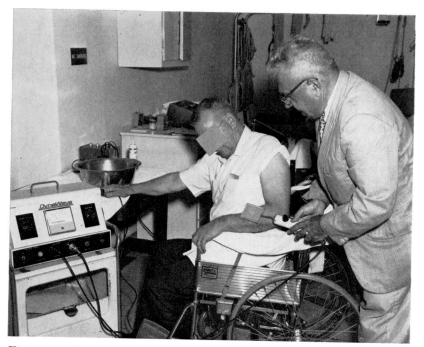

Figure 44. Sherrington's law of reciprocal innervation: Stimulation of agonists (i.e. here the wrist extensors) causes the relaxation of antagonists (i.e. here, the spastic wrist flexors).

him to attempt to raise his arm, extend the elbow, and extend the wrist and fingers whenever he feels the current, i.e. with each stimulus, as it is not so much the stimulation that is important, as the effort which the patient makes.

In order to conserve therapist's time, I tried to see if he or she could be replaced by a mechanical reminder to the patient. To accomplish this, I had a buzzer inserted in the circuit, so that every time the muscles were stimulated a buzzing sound was produced. (Fig. 46 shows the setup with the buzzer on the table.) It proved to be unsatisfactory. Even with the buzzer loud enough to disturb the therapist, the patient still was inclined to forget to try and perform the motions. Perhaps a loud speaker attachment, calling for him to raise his arm might have worked better. It is my considered opinion that S. A. E., if it is to work at all, requires

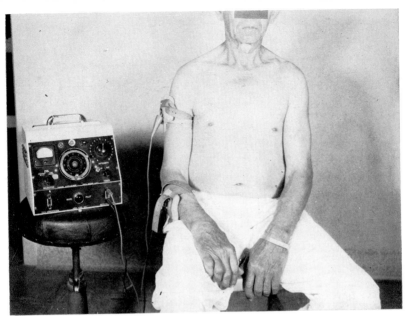

Figure 45. a. *(this page) and b.* show patient receiving S.A.E. routine, followed by pulley exercises, c. to g., to maintain range of motion (R.O.M.).

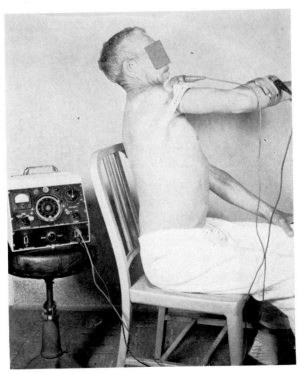

Figure 45b.

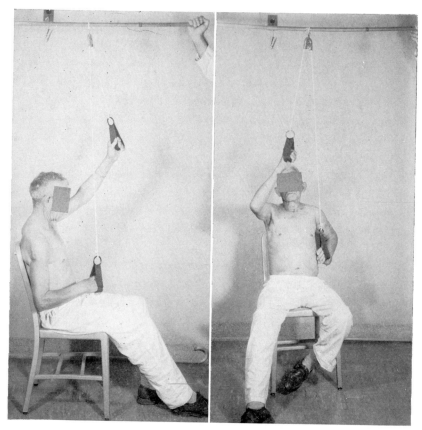

Figure 45c. *(left)* and d. *(right).*

a therapist or a therapy assistant or even a volunteer, to stand by the patient and remind him to attempt the exercise each time that he feels the current.

Following the treatment, the electrodes are removed, and the patient is encouraged to perform pulley exercise to maintain

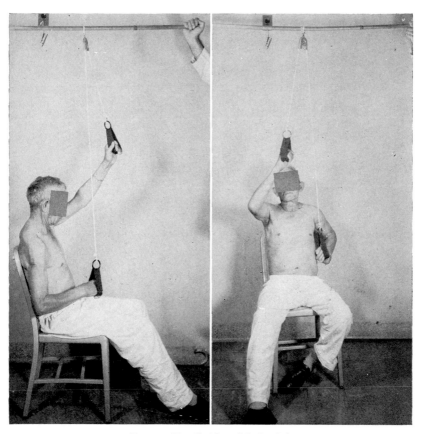

Figure 45e. *(left)* and f. *(right)*.

the range of motion (Fig. 45 c to g). If occupational therapy is available, it should also be encouraged, such as sanding or polishing, using the nonparetic hand to assist the paretic hand with the exercise. S.A.E. should be continued for at least three months, and longer, if there is any sign of progress. Even a partially func-

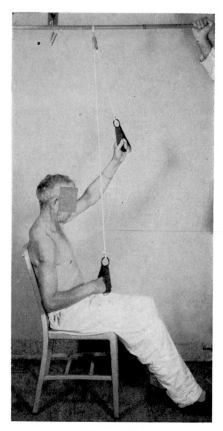

Figure 45g.

tioning upper extremity is better than a completely nonfunction-
ing one. If a rehabilitation therapy assistant or a member of the
family is available, S.A.E. can be continued as long as necessary,
even when the patient is discharged to home, when a member
of his family can be trained to supervise the treatment.

Another nice feature of this S.A.E. routine is that one therapist
can supervise one or more patients, either treated by different
stimulators (Fig. 47) or by one stimulator with the patients in
series (Fig. 48 a and b).

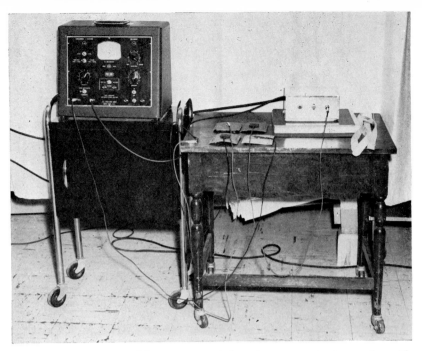

Figure 46. Buzzer on table top to remind patient to contract muscles with each stimulus.

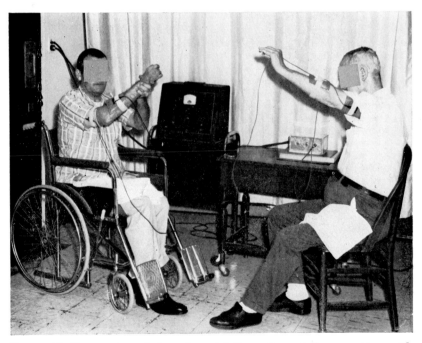

Figure 47. Two patients being given S.A.E. routine, at the same time with two sinusoidal stimulators.

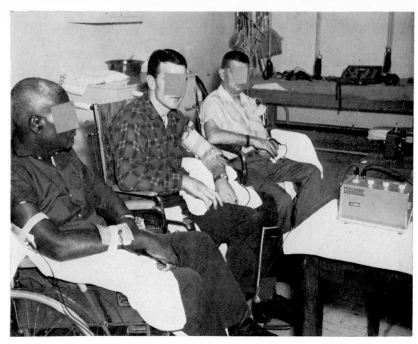

Figure 48, a and b. Three patients, connected in series, being given S.A.E. routine, with *one* stimulator. a. *(this page)*. Before stimulation.

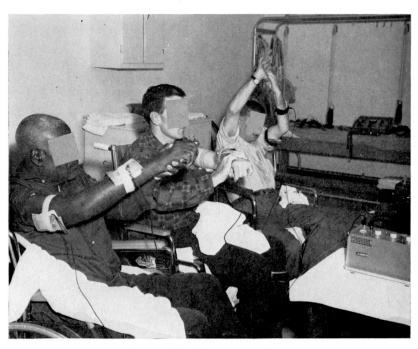

Figure 48b. During stimulation.

SUMMARY

While the paralyzed upper extremity does not as a rule recover its function to the same extent as the lower extremity, nevertheless a good rehabilitation program requires that efforts be made to promote such recovery. Passive exercise, active assistive exercise, and various types of special techniques should be undertaken, consistent with the training of members of the rehabilitation team. S.A.E. routine, which can be administered even at home by non-trained personnel, under appropriate supervision, merits consideration when further improvement is desired, if there has been some return of function in a paralyzed spastic upper extremity.

ADDENDUM

While S.A.E. was developed primarily for the restoration of function of upper extremity paralysis, it is not limited to the upper extremity. S.A.E. can be given just as profitably for lower extremity paralysis, where the patient has some voluntary function and needs neuromuscular reeducation. The application of stimulation to the hip and knee extensors, and ankle dorsiflexors while the patient attempts to contract these muscles should help with recovery of function in the lower extremity. A final reminder: patients following a stroke, should not be expected to remember to carry out a routine by themselves. A therapist or aide, a volunteer, or a member of his family should always be present to encourage and remind the patient to attempt to carry out the proper exercises, as he feels the current stimulus.

CRITIQUE OF S.A.E.

As every researcher knows, claims made for results of a treatment are not of much value unless adequate controls are used. In my original research on S.A.E., the patients were their own controls. I submitted my results to a psychologist statistician who concluded that they were statistically significant, namely p was less than 0.001. However, I still would like to see some center or group undertake a research project in which S.A.E. would be compared to other methods of treatment, particularly with active assistive exercise and with no treatment at all. I would predict that S.A.E. would give the best results, provided someone stayed with the patients and reminded them to try to contract their muscles with each stimulus.

Chapter 13

DYSKINESIA (DYSSYNERGY)

I N addition to the paresis on the hemiplegic side and the milder weakness on the so-called uninvolved or nonparetic limbs, another type of dyskinesia is often seen. This disturbance of movement occurs primarily where the C.V.A. involves the blood supply to the cerebellum, or its connections, i.e. the superior, anterior, inferior, or posterior cerebellar arteries. This neocerebellar syndrome, as described by Holmes[40] and Peele,[41] is characterized by homolateral atonia, disorders of muscular contraction, disorders of voluntary movement, and tremor. The overall term for the disturbed motion is *incoordination* or *dyssynergy*.

When equilibritory muscular activity is disturbed, then we have *dysequilibrium,* during attempted standing, or walking. When the disturbance involves nonequilibratory movement, we call it *ataxia* or *asynergy.*

The various manifestations of ataxia are, (a) dysmetria, or an increased amount of movement necessary to reach an object, and (b) decomposition of movement, which refers to the breakdown of a combined motion, such as of the shoulder, elbow, wrist, and fingers into its various individual components.

Other examples of this asynergy may be seen when the patient tries to sit up from the recumbent position, or to touch the examiners hand with his toes, or to kneel on a chair, or in the finger-to-nose test, or heel-to-knee test. In each of these cases, the patient performs the task by individualizing the various joint movements, and overshooting or undershooting the mark. When the patient is asked to grasp an object, or quickly to reverse the outstretched hand from the prone to the supine position, the same dysmetria can be elicited.

The inability to execute alternating and successive movements rapidly and smoothly, as for example, playing pat-a-cake, is called

120

adiadochokinesis or *dysdiadochokinesis.* Another manifestation of dysmetria is the rebound phenomenon. For example, the patient is asked by the examiner to extend the flexed forearm against resistance, and as the examiner suddenly releases the resistance, the patient's hand will shoot out. All of these symptoms are seen when there is unilateral cerebellar involvement, in which case, the symptoms above described occur on the side of the lesion. Two other manifestations of cerebellar involvement are asthenia and atony.

TREATMENT

The treatment of dysequilibrium and ataxia should be directed to the respective manifestations. Dysequilibrium requires frequent practice between parallel bars of standing and walking. Only when the patient has shown that he can negotiate the bars without holding on is he allowed to progress to crutch and later to cane ambulation. For *ataxia,* for patients with no paralysis but poor coordination, we prescribe coordination exercises, which are as follows:

Group 1

1. Sit or recline on a rug or hard mattress, or plinth, both hips and knees extended, back supported by back rest.
2. Bend right hip and knee towards you, trying to keep heel in straight line.
3. Return to original position, again sliding heel in straight line.
4. and 5. Repeat 2 and 3 with left leg.
6. and 7. Repeat 2 and 3 with both legs.
8. Slide right heel sideways as far as you can.
9. Return to original position.
10. and 11. Repeat with left leg.
12. and 13. Repeat with both legs.
14. Bend right knee to 90 degrees.
15. Abduct leg, keeping heel on mat.
16. Return to original position.
17. and 18. Repeat with left leg.
19. and 20. Repeat with both legs.

Repeat the entire group of exercises every two hours, for one week or longer, until they are done with ease. Then advance to Group 2.

Group 2

First repeat the above exercises once, and add the following:
1. Same position as Group 1.
2. Bend right knee to 90 degrees; keep left knee straight.
3. Place right heel on left knee.
4. Return to original position.
5. Straighten right knee.
6, 7, 8, and 9. Repeat with left heel to right knee.

Repeat Group 2 every two hours for one or more weeks, until mastered.

Group 3

Repeat Group 1 and Group 2 once; then proceed to Group 3.
1. Bend right knee to 90 degrees.
2. Place right heel on left knee.
3. Return.
4. Place right heel on left ankle.
5. Return.
6. Place right heel on left knee.
7. Return.
8. Place right heel on left ankle.
9. Return.
10. to 18. Repeat 1 to 9 with left heel on right knee and ankle.
19. Now, alternate; bend right knee to 90 degrees.
20. Place right heel on left knee.
21. Return and straighten right knee.
22. Now bend left knee to 90 degrees.
23. Place left heel on right ankle.
24. Return and straighten left knee.

Do this exercise two times every two hours for one week or until mastered.

Group 4

Repeat exercise Groups 1, 2, and 3 once; then proceed to Group 4. Same position.
1. Place right heel on left knee.

2. Slide heel down leg to ankle.
3. Slide heel back to knee.
4. Return to original position.
5, 6, 7, and 8. Repeat with left heel on right knee.

Repeat exercise four times every two hours or until mastered (one or more weeks) and go to Group 5.

Group 5

Repeat exercise Groups 1 to 4 once; then proceed to Group 5.
1. Bend right knee. (Keep left knee straight.)
2. Extend right leg and bend left knee.
3. Abduct right leg and extend left leg.
4. Abduct left leg and bend right knee.
5. Bring both legs back to original position.

Repeat four times, three times a day until mastered.

Group 6

First mark each leg with red ink, as follows: Write number 1 on knees, number 2 over mid legs, and number 3 on ankles. The object is to place alternate heels on numbers 1, 2, and 3 as follows.

1. Place right heel on left 1.
2. Return.
3. Place left heel on right 1.
4. Return.
5. Place right heel on left 2.
6. Return.
7. Place left heel on right 2.
8. Return.
9. Place right heel on left 3.
10. Return.
11. Place left heel on right 3.
12. Return.

Now have a family member call out "right heel on left 2," "return," "left heel on right 3," "return," etc. Repeat four times, three times a day, until mastered.

Exercises to Promote Equilibrium—Standing to Sitting and Reverse

Sitting Exercises

1. Patient stands between parallel bars, or in the absence of parallel bars, holds onto the back of a chair, which has to be stable.
2. Place a chair behind patient.
3. Instruct patient to sit down in chair, slowly.
4. Instruct patient to stand up slowly.

Caution patient to keep body slightly forward in sitting down or standing up. Repeat every two hours, four times, for one week or longer if necessary.

Walking Exercise (a)

1. Draw a line on floor in center of, and parallel to, parallel bars.
2. Have patient stand at the beginning of the parallel bars, holding on to them if necessary.
3. Ask patient to walk, from one end of bars to the other, keeping each foot three inches from center line.
4. Have patient turn around and return.

Repeat four times and rest.

Walking Exercise (b)

Repeat 1 to 4 without the patient holding onto the parallel bars. When the patient has mastered this, then proceed to walking exercise (c).

Walking Exercise (c)

Draw a line on the floor and have the patient repeat without holding on to anything, but stay with him in case of loss of equilibrium.

Every day start with sitting down and getting up and then proceed to walking. If necessary, the patient may use a cane or crutch until his confidence in walking is restored. After the patient has overcome his dysequilibrium and if he needs further practice in walking, but is still too weak, the routine then will be as in the hemiplegic intermittent double step gait as described by Peszczynski:[31] Step forward with the stronger leg and cane; bring the weaker foot to the side of the stronger foot; rest. Lean slightly forward and repeat.

Chapter 14

DYSKINESIA: SPASTICITY

ONE of the problems that interferes with the patient's rehabilitation following a stroke is spasticity. True, in certain cases some spasticity can be helpful. For example, a certain amount of spasticity in the paretic quadriceps helps to keep the knee in extention during the stance phase of ambulation, and thus assists the patient with walking or standing. At the same time, however, the usual concomitant spasticity of the triceps surae combined with the weakness of the ankle dorsiflexors results in a contracture of the gastrocnemius, prevents the patient from putting the foot on the ground, and causes him to drag his foot and walk on his toes. Furthermore, this combination of spasticity of the quadriceps and of the calf muscles is frequently manifested by marked clonus, thus interfering with ambulation altogether.

In the upper extremity, on the other hand, spasticity has no redeeming value at all. The usual picture of the spastic upper extremity consists of adduction of the shoulder, forward flexion of the arm, flexion of the elbow, pronation of the forearm, flexion of the wrist with ulnar deviation, flexion of the fingers and thumb, sometimes so severe that the nails dig into the flesh. Furthermore, spasticity is a hindrance to rehabilitation because a spastic muscle, even if only partially paralyzed, prevents contraction of its antagonists, again interfering with function. Thus, it is often necessary to try to reduce spasticity if excessive, or to eliminate it altogether. Before discussing the various ways of treating spasticity with a view to its elimination, let us review some of the basic features.

Spasticity may be defined as a condition of voluntary muscle which resists passive stretching. The clinical manifestation of spasticity are (a) increased resistance to stretch, (b) increased reflexes, and (c) clonus. Next follows a brief review of the anatomy of voluntary muscle.

126

SALIENT ANATOMY OF VOLUNTARY MUSCLE

Voluntary muscle is composed of two types of muscle fibers, intrafusal and extrafusal. The intrafusal muscle fibers combine to form a muscle spindle which is a fibrous capsule a few millimeters in length that lies to one side of a muscle fasciculus.[42] In the middle of the spindle is the "nuclear bag," consisting of a noncontracting area composed of muscle nuclei. Surrounding the muscle spindles are the extrafusal muscle fibers. Each extrafusal muscle fiber is a large multinucleated cell varying in length from one to forty-one millimeters, and in thickness from ten to one hundred micra.[43] The muscle spindles have receptor organs from which sensory impulses are carried to the central nervous system by afferent nerve fibers. From the central nervous system efferent impulses are carried to the intrafusal fibers by efferent nerve fibers called *gamma fibers*. The extrafusal muscle fibers, on the other hand, are stimulated by different efferent fibers from the spinal cord—the *alpha* motor fibers. Two additional sensory pathways should be mentioned. One is the sensory nerves carrying impulses from receptors situated where muscle fibers insert into the tendon. These are so-called Golgi tendon organ receptors. And finally, nerve endings in the skin also carry impulses, pain, touch, heat and cold, to the central nervous system.

The afferent impulses from the muscle spindles are carried to the central nervous system by fibers which can be classified as group (1a) and group (2). The (1a) fibers form a direct monosynaptic connection with the alpha motor neuron in the anterior horn of the spinal cord. The group (2) fibers on the other hand, reach the lateral or intermediate horn of the spinal cord and form multisynaptic connections with the anterior horn cells. The (1b) fibers arise from the Golgi tendon organ receptors and form duosynaptic connection with the anterior horn cells of their muscle and its synergists. In addition to the alpha fibers in the motor neuron, as previously described, are the gamma fibers, stimulation of which produces a contraction of the intrafusal muscle fibers with stretching of the nuclear bag and stimulation of the (1a) fibers.

Upper Motor Neurons

Fibers from different parts of the brain descend in the lateral or intermediate columns of the spinal cord, and form synaptic connections with the anterior horn cells. These fibers coming from the higher centers have a facilitory or inhibitory effect on the anterior horn cells, but mostly inhibitory. Thus, if there is some interference with these impulses, the result is muscle spasticity, primarily because of the gamma motor neurons which normally are inhibited, and now, by release of these inhibitions, become overactive, although, as Takamari,[44] has shown, independent facilitation of the spinal alpha motor neuron also occurs.

SPASTICITY

Physiologically speaking, therefore, *spasticity may be described as an overactivity of gamma motor neurons due to the loss of inhibition from the brain.* This loss of inhibition is one of the usual manifestations of a stroke. In order to overcome this spasticity, it is necessary to reduce the overactivity of the gamma motor neurons. This reduction of overactivity should be just enough to diminish or eliminate the spasticity and yet not so much as to interfere with motor function. We shall now discuss the various procedures that have been used in the past, and indicate what we believe is a possibility for the future treatment of this deterrent to rehabilitation.

Treatment of Spasticity

Physical Treatment

HEAT. The application of heat to spastic muscle, either by infrared or luminous heat, by short or microwave diathermy, or by hydrocollator pack, will cause muscular relaxation while the heat is applied and for a short period thereafter. Application of general heat as by a Hubbard tank, or Moistaire Cabinet, or by a horizontal whirlpool will have a similar temporary effect.

COLD. The application of cold directly on the muscle or nerve, whether by ice water or by a hydrocollator cold pack, will also result in a temporary reduction of spasticity. This is probably, as Zankel has shown,[45] because of a reduction of nerve conduction velocity. Khalili[43] postulates that this may be a result of the in-hibitory effect on the afferent impulses from the skin.

COLD AND HEAT. Tigney and Sheldon[46] applied heat to the nonparetic parts of the body and cold to the spastic muscles. In the cat, such treatment was shown by Newton and Lehmkuhl[47] to reduce muscle spindle activity.

COOLING OF THE SPINAL CORD. Negrin[48] cooled the spinal sub-dural and subarachnoid space by laminectomy and perfusion, or by catheter insertion, with long-lasting relief of spasticity and without impairment of sensation or motor power. The probable explanation is the reduction of impulses from the anterior horn cells to the intrafusal fibers.

SINUSOIDAL STIMULATION. Lee[49] stimulated the spastic muscles to the point of fatigue and succeeded in reducing spasticity temporarily. And according to Sherrington's well-known law of reciprocal innervation, "Stimulation of Agonists causes a relaxa-tion of antagonists," Zankel[39] in his S.A.E. routine stimulated by a *sinusoidal current* the extensors of the elbow, wrist, and fingers to cause a temporary reduction in flexor spasticity to allow the patient to use any latent power in the extensors to overcome the flexors.

Stretching of the spastic muscle will mechanically overcome the spasticity, again only temporarily.

ULTRASOUND. In studying the effect of various physical modali-ties on nerve conduction velocity, pallesthesia, and nerve tempera-ture,[45] it was noted that cold, compression, and ultrasound all had the same effect on nerve conduction velocity, namely a re-duction. It was thought therefore, that these modalities might have an effect on spasticity. Cold was discussed above. Com-pression, no doubt, would have such an effect, but would also interfere with the circulation. But ultrasound applied to the nerve and/or muscle seemed worthwhile trying, as a safe proce-dure. In our clinic numerous patients presented themselves with varying degrees of spasticity and seemed ideal subjects for an attempt at clinical evaluation of this disabling condition. We started with mild ultrasonation, namely one watt per square centimeter for five minutes. A dynamometer was used to measure the resistance to stretch before and after treatment. An electromyograph was used to study the motor unit activity during stretch before and after ultrasound. Early results seem promising. It is postulated that application of ultrasound of the right frequency, strength, and duration will reduce spasticity without too much interference with motion or sensation.

It is suggested that before trying radical surgical procedures or even chemical injections into nerve or muscle, ultrasound be applied daily to the involved nerve, three watts per square centimeter, for fifteen minutes, for one month, or longer if preliminary results warrant. Figure 49 shows ultrasound applied to posterior tibial nerve for spastic triceps surae.

Chemical Treatment

DRUGS. In recent years numerous drugs have been prescribed for so-called spasm of skeletal muscle following strain. While

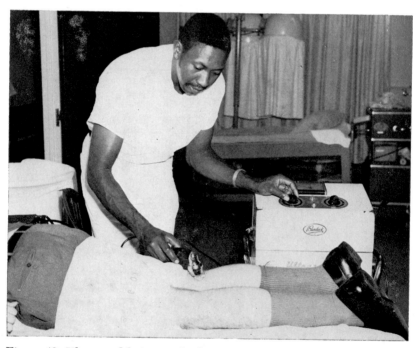

Figure 49. Ultrasound being applied to posterior tibial nerve in an attempt to reduce spasticity of spastic triceps surae.

they may succeed in this function, they seem to have no effect at all on spasticity in stroke patients. This author was privileged to try Valium®(diazepam) when still in the experimental stage for the attempted relief of spasticity in paraplegia. Unfortunately, the amount necessary to produce any results so weakened the patient that he could not carry out any activity whatsoever. Similarly, d-tubocurarine has been used for relief of spasticity by blocking the myoneural junction. Again, while spasticity is reduced, voluntary power is concomitantly diminished.

CHEMICAL INJECTIONS. Recently certain chemical agents have come into increasing use in the treatment of spasticity. These include procaine into nerve, cord, or muscle; phenol into nerve, muscle, or spinal cord; alcohol into muscle and nerve,[42] with reportedly good results but with some unwanted side effects.

Surgical Treatment

Surgical methods that have been used for relief of spasticity include: (a) section of the anterior nerve roots (anterior rhizotomy), (b) section of the posterior nerve roots, (posterior rhizotomy), (c) section of the cord (cordotomy), (d) section of the nerve (neurectomy), and (e) section of the tendon (tenotomy). In careful hands these procedures have proven effective for relief of spasticity.

Chapter 15

DYSESTHESIA (ANESTHESIA)– (HYPESTHESIA)

As is well known, patients suffering from C.V.A.'s not only manifest paralysis of one side of the body, but very often have disturbed sensation in the paretic limbs. What is not generally realized is that the sensory involvement often is greater than the motor involvement and, just as is true of the motor involvement in the nonparetic limbs, so also there may be sensory disturbances in the same, i.e. nonparetic, limbs. Loss of, or abnormal, sensation is called *dysesthesia*.

Dysesthesias in stroke patients take many forms. We shall now review some of these and indicate the possible causes and management of these sensory difficulties.

The usual disturbance in sensation following a stroke is hemianesthesia, or the loss of, or reduced, sensation on the same side as the paresis, i.e. opposite the locale of the C.V.A. and a partial loss of sensation on the homolateral side. The patient will often describe his symptoms as *numbness*, and if he is alert, he will also indicate that he has lost power to perceive touch, pain, heat, or cold. These sensations can be tested by the examiner, who will often find that the sensation is not lost, but diminished, and that some of these sensations will be retained, while others are lost. Too, sometimes the examiner will note a reversal of the sense of heat and cold, the patient calling "heat," "cold," and "cold," "heat." Sometimes the hemianesthesia is alternating (attributed to involvement of pons or medulla), and as already noted, the loss of sensation is usually nontotal, as each hemisphere of the brain receives some sensory impulses from both sides of the body, just as is true of motor innervation.

Many of these patients suffer from inability to appreciate

double simultaneous stimuli–called *extinction*. The test is as follows:

1. Tell patient to close his eyes.
2. Press two cotton swabs firmly over two opposite areas of the body, i.e. two arms, two legs, two thighs.
3. Ask patient to point to the areas of contact–"Put your finger on the spot where I am touching you."
4. Note the response. Frequently the patient will point to only one area, thus showing that he is suffering from *extinction*.

Bilateral homonomous hemianopsia, causing blindness in one half of each eye, is a common symptom following a stroke. This is tested by having the patient and examiner face one another, the patient closing one eye at a time while an object is held to one side and gradually brought into view. Assuming that the examiner has normal vision, he will be the first to perceive the object. The degree of hemianopsia will be determined by the distance it takes for the patient to see the object after the examiner has seen it. In homonomous hemianopsia, (or hemianopia) the loss of vision is in the right or left half of both eyes, i.e. on the same side as the hemiplegia. This disturbance in vision will affect the patient's rehabilitation unless the Rehabilitation Team recognizes it and acts accordingly. The more detailed program has been discussed under progressive rehabilitation phases. But at this time, suffice it to say that all activity to be meaningful to the patient must be directed from the side at which normal vision prevails.

Among other forms of dysesthesia should be mentioned *anosmia*, or loss of sense of smell. Since the olfactory nerves send sensory impulses to both sides of the brain, loss of the sense of smell is not perceived by the patient in unilateral disease. To test for the sense of smell, one must therefore use various fragrant substances applied to each nostril separately. Irritation of the cortical center for smell will result in *parosmia*, or hallucinations of smell.

Loss of the sensation of taste also is not common in stroke patients. When it occurs, unless each side of the tongue is tested separately, it will be missed. Such loss, if present, is called *ageusia*. Diminished sensation of taste is *hypogeusia*, and hallucinations of taste are called *parageusia*. The sensation of hearing and seeing will best be discussed under Dysphasia, Chapter 16. There remains to be considered the peripheral sensation for vibration or *pallesthesia*. Because we had available an instrument with which we could study this sensation quantitatively, we shall now consider it in more detail.

A pallesthesiometer is an instrument that measures vibrations in terms of microns of motion. It is a *quantitative tuning fork*. By means of such an instrument (Bio-thesiometer—Biomedical Instrument Company, Chagrin Falls, Ohio), forty stroke patients were examined as to their sensation for vibration in the forehead, upper lids, lower lids, cheek bones, mastoids, trunk, and upper and lower extremities (Fig. 50; see Zankel[50]). We found that vibratory sensation in the trunk and head showed no statistical significant differences between the paretic and nonparetic sides. In the extremities, however, of the forty patients tested, eleven had a normal sensation for vibration in the *paretic upper* ex-

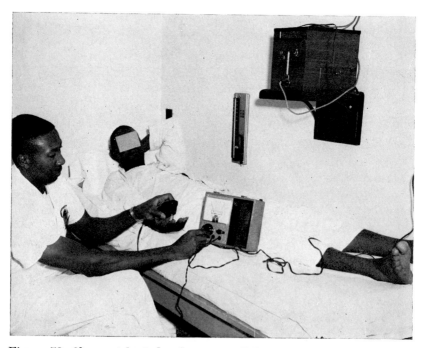

Figure 50. Shows right index finger tested for sensation of vibration by means of a pallesthesiometer.

tremity, and nine, in the *paretic lower* extremity. This would indicate that loss of motion and loss of sensation do not necessarily go together. Twenty-nine patients did have a diminished sensation for vibration *(pallhypesthesia)* or complete loss of sensation *(pallanesthesia)* in the paretic extremities, and some loss of sensation in the nonparetic extremities. Furthermore, twenty-three patients who recovered their motor function in the upper and lower extremities were studied as to their recovery from the diminished vibratory sense. Of these, fifteen had a persistent pallhypesthesia in the previously paretic upper extremity, and twenty-one, in the previously paretic lower extremity. Such residual pallhypesthesia in patients who had had a stroke and who had made a good motor functional recovery will explain their inability to cooperate with their rehabilitation program. An attempt was made to improve this vibratory sense by the use of sinusoidal stimulation to the palm and sole, and the results were promising. The explanation would be the same as was the case with the S.A.E. routine, i.e. stimulation helped to develop new pathways to sensory areas of the brain.[39]

Figures 51 a, b, c, 52, and 53 show technic of stimulation to improve sensation for vibration.

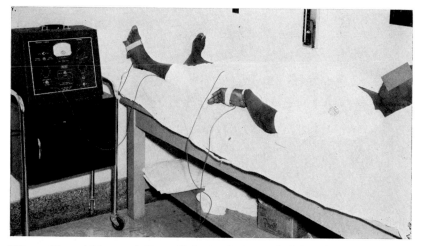

Figure 51. a. *(this page)* Sinusoidal stimulation to left hand and left foot in an attempt to improve sensation for vibration.

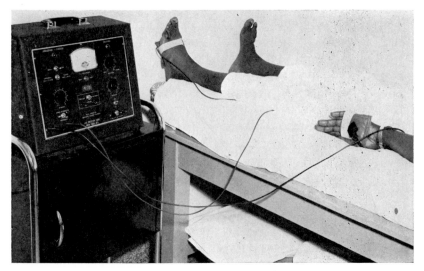

Figure 51b. Close up view of same.

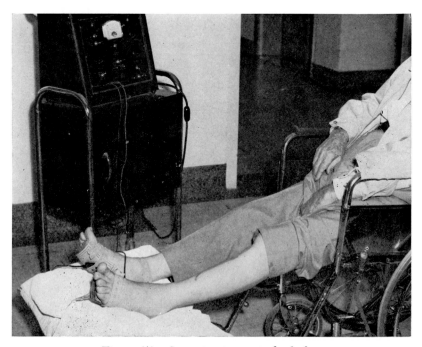

Figure 51c. Same treatment to both feet.

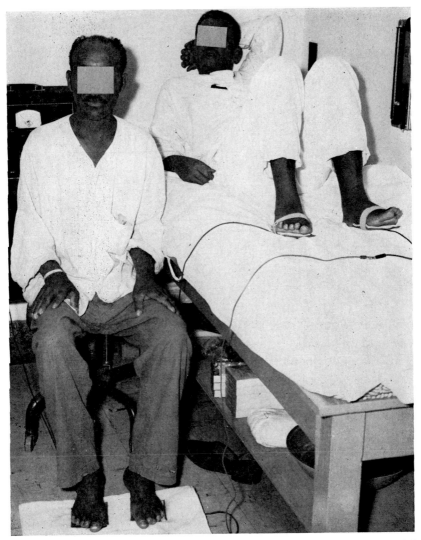

Figure 52. Both feet of two patients, in series, being treated by sinusoidal stimulation, in order to improve sensation for vibration.

DYSESTHESIA—PAINFUL SENSATION

So far we have considered loss of sensation or diminished sensation following a stroke. We shall now discuss some of the abnormal sensations.

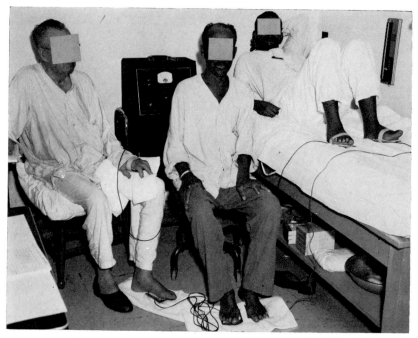

Figure 53. Three patients, in series, being treated by one stimulator; patient on left has electrodes under left hand and left foot; while the other two patients have electrodes under both feet.

Thalamic Pain

Several weeks after the onset of a stroke, the patient develops pain in the paretic side. The pain is of a burning type and is usually worse in the extremities, particularly the hand. This burning pain may persist for months. Thalamic crying is often associated with this pain. The treatment is tranquilization. If severe, it may require destruction of various parts of the thalamus by electrocautery, ultrasound, or freezing.

Shoulder-Hand Syndrome

Again, several weeks after a stroke, there frequently develops pain in the shoulder radiating down the arm and hand. The usual cause of this is disuse. The pain is often accompanied by a shoulder subluxation, manifested by a definite space between the tuberosity of the humerus and acromion process of the scapula.

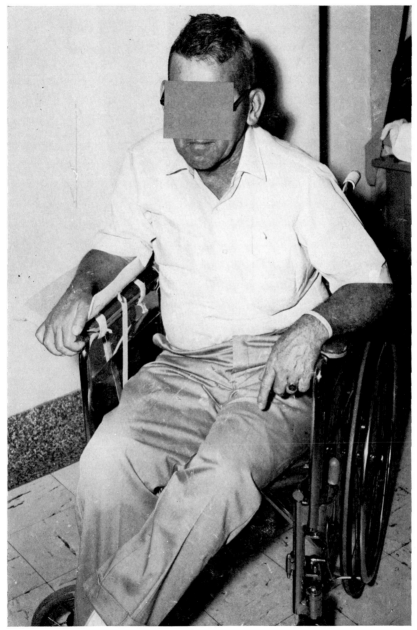

Figure 54. Shows patient's rt arm resting on homemade padded shell attached to rt arm of wheelchair.

The best treatment is *prevention* by active exercise if possible, or by passive exercise including sinusoidal stimulation if necessary. It is also important to keep the shoulder in a sling and not to let it hang when the patient walks. When he sits, it is desirable to provide his wheelchair with an arm rest, upon which the patient will keep his forearm whenever he does not use it for self-care activities. (Figs. 54 to 57 show the patient resting the paretic arm on a home-made padded half-shell attached to the arm of a wheelchair. Fig. 54 shows overall view, and Figs. 55, 56, and 57 show a close-up view.)

The treatment for painful shoulder is the application of a hot wet pack for thirty minutes, followed by sedative massage and active or passive exercise. If no relief is obtained in a reasonable time, ultrasound, one to two watts per square centimeter applied

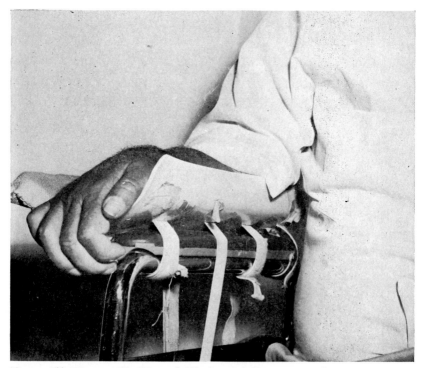

Figure 55. Figures 55, 56, and 57 show close-up view of same arm rest. (Note: We find this more comfortable than having patient's arm constantly in shoulder sling.)

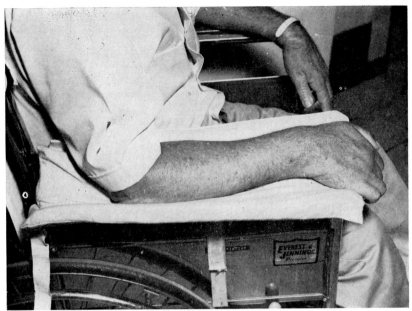

Figure 56.

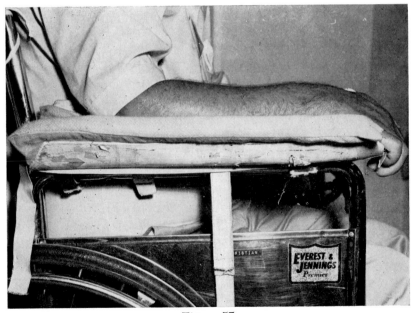

Figure 57.

to the shoulder for five minutes will often give relief. For persistent, severe pain, surgical treatment will have to be considered, such as arthrodesis of the glenohumeral joint.

Chapter 16

DYSPHASIA (APHASIA)

DEFINITION

DYSPHASIA (aphasia) is a disturbance in communication manifested by an inability to comprehend or to express language symbols. In the present monograph we are limiting our discussion to such impairment associated with stroke and more specifically with centers in the brain which have to do with comprehension and/or expression.

INCIDENCE

It is generally agreed that dysphasia is invariably associated with right hemiplegia, that is, left-sided brain damage. Wepman[51] quotes Alexander Louria, that in an investigation of 394 brain injured patients in Moscow, not one case of right brain damage and aphasia was noted. Where a left hemiplegia shows manifestations of speech involvement, closer observation will reveal them to be disturbances in language skills, i.e. dysarthria, rather than dysphasia as above defined. By dysarthia we mean the loss of use of, or diminished strength or coordination of speech production musculature.

In our own series of 500 patients,[52] we found 199 patients with dysphasia (39.8%); of these 167 (93.4%) were primarily expressive; 18 (3.6%) were primarily receptive, and 14 (2.8%) were of the mixed or combined type.

TESTING FOR DYSPHASIA

Numerous tests have been developed for delineating the type and degree of dysphasia. Where a speech pathologist or speech therapist is available, some of these tests can be very helpful. For example, The Language Modalities Test for Aphasia by Wepman and Jones[53] presents a balanced set of tests which require the patient to show his auditory, oral, visual, and graphic abilities.

Schuel *et al.*[54] employ the Minnesota Test for Differential Diagnosis of Aphasia, which they designed to help determine whether the aphasia in a patient is reversible.

Porch[55] in his Porch Index of Communicative abilities, means to provide prognostic information. Jon Eisenson has developed a series of tests, embodied in a record form for use with Chapter VI of his manual *Examining for Aphasia.*[56]

CLASSIFICATION

Based upon sophisticated testing such as mentioned above, the speech pathologist can indicate to the physician the specific type of dysphasia from which the patient is suffering, and he can outline the treatment which can be given by the speech therapist, if available, or by other medical personnel, and even by the family. In our own hospital, (Veterans Administration Hospital, Columbia, South Carolina), when for many years we had no speech pathologist or therapist, the following outline helped the P. M. and R. and nursing personnel to deal with this important and often difficult problem. Our simplified classification of the types of aphasia is as follows:

1. Sensory or receptive or evaluative.
    a. Auditory aphasia—inability to comprehend the meaning of various sounds.
    b. Visual aphasia—inability to comprehend visible characters.
2. Motor or expressive or productive dysphasia (verbal apraxia)
    a. Anomia—inability to give names of objects or of subjects.
    b. Agraphia—inability to produce graphic symbols, i.e. to write meaningfully.
    c. Acalculia—inability to do simple arithmetic.
    d. Paraphasia—inability to express continuous thoughts, manifested by transposition of symbols, words, or letters.
    e. Dysprosody—inability to speak with variable speech or rhythm manifested by a monotonous type of speech.
3. Mixed dysphasia, combining both receptive and expressive types.

MANAGEMENT OF THE PATIENT WITH DYSPHASIA

Where a speech pathologist or speech therapist is available, he will institute treatment and guide the other members of the rehabilitation team to carry on in his absence. Where such a trained individual is not available, the following guide may be of some help to nursing and other rehabilitation personnel.

Principles of Treatment

1. Determine the patient's background, education, work history, and hobbies. Use this background in your communication with patient.
2. Remember that the basis for communication is auditory stimulation combined with visual stimulation.
3. To be effective, these stimuli should be intense, clear, repetitive, and slow.
4. Encourage the patient to respond. Do not force, be patient; do not push, pull.
5. Encourage the patient to communicate, if only with gestures, and with physical response to commands.
6. As the patient progresses in recovery from dysphasia, gradually withdraw the auditory impulses and continue with visual impulses.
7. Motivate the patient by complementing him; do not criticize.

Objectives

The members of the nursing staff, and the PM&R personnel and/or the family should be made aware by the speech pathologist, speech therapist, or by the patient's physician of the therapeutic goals. These are as follows:

1. To develop understandable speech.
2. To develop reading, spelling skills, and writing with the nonparetic extremity, if necessary.
3. To provide opportunities for self-expression.
4. To aid the patient to accept himself in the light of his present situation.
5. To help the patient to develop emotional balance.
6. To avoid frustrating situations, so as to minimize the incidence of anxiety.

In applying the above principles and objectives, the following suggestions may be helpful to the nurse, nursing assistant, and other allied professional personnel, including PM&R personnel, and the members of the family.

1. Treat the patient like the grown-up that he is. Remember, he may be aphasic, but he is not a child.

2. Communicate with the patient by the use of every day surroundings. "You look cold; let me help you with your sweater," or "It's kind of hot; let's put on the fan or the air conditioner," as the case may be. "Here's an apple," or a pear or any other fruit or food.

3. Do not criticize the patient if he can not say something that he said before. Just because he mentioned your name yesterday does not mean that he can necessarily say it today. Do not remind him of his past accomplishments in a critical manner, but in a friendly way repeat your name or whatever word he used and give him a chance to say it if he wants to and if he can.

4. Let your language be simple. Use everyday words. Give him a chance to answer your questions with a "yes or "no." Remember, however, that often a patient will answer "yes" when he really means "no," or vice versa.

5. Do not become irritable or impatient if your patient cannot indicate with gestures what he cannot verbalize or write. But explore these different ways to communicate.

6. Be aware that one of the symptoms of a stroke patient is perseveration, where the patient repeats the same word or act, or impersistence, where the patient cannot concentrate on an act, or view, or sound. In other words, his attention span is poor. This symptom in a stroke patient is not often recognized.

7. Also, do not be horrified if the patient uses four-letter words. You do not have to repeat them, just ignore them, and carry on as if he did not say them.

8. Speak slowly, and with a voice loud enough to be heard by the patient, but do not shout, unless the patient happens to be hard-of-hearing.

9. Use letters and figures that are large enough for the patient to see, and if he needs glasses, by all means, make sure that he gets them.

10. Finally, let your attitude always be hopeful. Sometimes, after months of apparent failure, the patient will suddenly make sense even if his vocabulary remains limited.

DISCUSSION

Elaine Sands and co-workers[57] studied thirty patients who had aphasia due to C.V.A. at a median age of 56.5 years and who had received speech therapy. They followed them four to twelve months after the termination of therapy. They examined changes in scores on what they called Functional Communication Profile (F.C.P.) with relation to age, time before onset of treatment, time in treatment, amount of treatment, and severity of impairment. Their conclusions were as follows: (a) Significant improvement in language function often occurs after the first year following a stroke (b) Patients under fifty have a better chance of recovery than those over sixty.

In our own experience[52] and at my request, an analysis by a qualified speech therapist at the Veterans Administration Hospital, Columbia, South Carolina of one hundred patients with dysphasia showed that 10 percent profited by her treatment to the point where she could see definite improvement. In 90 percent of the patients, the improvement was so slight as for me to question the need for a speech therapist. When the therapist resigned, I did not ask for a replacement. This does not mean that intensive speech therapy should not be tried where a trained therapist is available and where suitable financial arrangements can be made for such treatment. But for the stroke patients with dysphasia, it would seem that subprofessional personnel in hospitals and nursing care centers and even the members of the family, where the patient is at home, can be the mainstay of such treatment. It should be noted here, however, that we are referring to strokes resulting from cerebrovascular accidents. Dysphasias resulting from traumatic or operative hemiplegias are another matter. Patients suffering from dysphasia due to these causes, especially in the younger age group, can definitely be helped by a professional speech therapy program.

DYSPHASIA GUIDE TO THE MEMBERS OF THE REHABILITATION TEAM

1. You can help with the retraining of the dysphasic patients by using common objects, every day items that the patient is familiar with. If you have the object, show it to him; if not, show him a good picture of the object.
2. Place the object in its proper perspective; for example, "Put your spoon in your soup." "The phone is ringing." "Can you see the phone?" "That's the phone ringing."
3. The therapist should calmly and intimately explain the ongoing procedure. "I'm now going to give you a massage to your wrist." "I'm putting a hot pack to your shoulder. It isn't going to be too hot. You see I'm trying it on myself." The occupational therapist says, "Let's do some sanding," and she shows the items.
4. Start early, and teach as you treat.
5. Finally, in rehabilitation of patients with right hemiplegia and dysphasia, it is good to remember that they have difficulty with *symbolic* language and even with simple arithmetic. On the other hand, patients with left hemiplegia have difficulty, not with symbols, but with *perceptual tasks*. They also have less appreciation of position of objects in space and of reproduction of what they see. Therefore, in retraining patients with right hemiplegia and dysphasia use language forms; show what you mean; use pantomime instruction. Point to the object. In retraining patients with left hemiplegia, use arithmetical and language symbols. Figure 58 shows a speech therapy trainee with a group of dysphasic patients.

TESTS FOR PROGNOSIS IN DYSPHASIA

As already noted above, Schuel[54] uses the Minnesota Test for Aphasia to determine if the dysphasia is reversible. A different prognostic test has been developed by Liberson[58] who stimulated the contraletal median nerve in patients with right hemiplegia and aphasia, and studied the evoked E.E.G. potentials, bilaterally, from central, parietal, and occipital regions, and found them suppressed, or completely depressed in ten of fifteen aphasic patients

on the involved side of the brain. He suggests that this test, therefore, promises to be of objective prognostic significance in speech
rehabilitation.

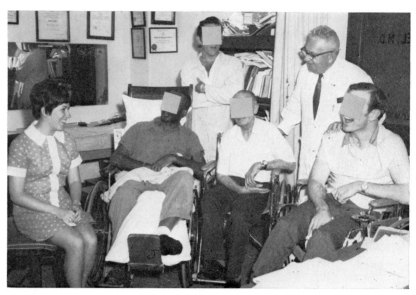

Figure 58. Shows a speech therapy trainee with a group of dysphasic
patients, author observing.

Chapter 17

DYSMENTIA

By *dysmentia,* we mean the neurotic and/or psychotic manifestations in stroke patients, as part of the stroke syndrome.
We do not mean the symptoms associated with dysphasia, dyskinesia, or dysesthesia, although admittedly, it is sometimes difficult to separate them. Dysmentia in stroke patients takes several
forms. It is important to remember that these mental symptoms
often occur without marked disturbance in motion or sensation, or
even communication. This, however, is the exception rather than
the rule. Usually the mental symptoms are associated with other
evidences of stroke.

The usual findings are confusion of mind, inability to think, and
inability to remember. There is loss of emotional control, manifested by easy excitation. Impersistence is commonly found in
stroke patients. This is manifested by the patient's inability to
concentrate upon an object or upon the examiner. The patient
is thus unable to follow simple instructions. Hence in order to
promote a good rehabilitation result it is necessary for the doctor
or therapist to keep prodding the patient in order to hold his
attention. Sometimes this impersistence can lead to danger, as in
failure to put out a lighted match.

Another manifestation of dysmentia is perseveration, as is seen
in asking the patient to count from one to ten. He will start,
"one, two, three, four, five, six," and stop at one of the numbers
and repeat it, "six, six," and then go on. Or at home he will turn
on the gas on the gas range and then try to turn it on again.

Thalamic crying is a well-recognized manifestation of dysmentia. The patient will cry without tears at the slightest provocation,
such as hearing his wife's name or being complemented on his
progress. Loud rhythmic laughter is not so well known. One of
our patients following a left hemiplegia would laugh at the slight-

est remark. His laughter would ring through the entire floor, "Ho! Ho! Ho! Ho!" This lasted from the beginning of his stroke and persisted right through to his discharge.

Confusion is quite common following a stroke. The patient may be able to read and write. But in the act of reading or writing he will suddenly drift and lose his trend. So often a patient will not be able to identify his locale. When asked, "Where are you?" instead of replying that he is in a hospital in the appropriate city, he will say that he is in his home city. Whether these symptoms are entirely due to the stroke or whether they are activated by the stroke, can only be determined by a careful history from the family and friends. From our observation, these symptoms are more prevalent in patients with right hemiplegia and dysphasia, although they are not uncommon in those with left hemiplegia.

Reactive depression in stroke patients is not at all unusual. Its management is the same as reactive depression without stroke. The same is true of psychosis and psychoneurosis. However, mental deterioration that leads to determination of mental incompetency is difficult to manage. Patients that reach this stage of mental inadequacy become pure nursing care problems.

To evaluate quickly the patient's mental state, I use the following ten questions:

1. What is the name of this place, or where are you now?
2. Where is it located? In what city?
3. What is today's date?
4. What month is it?
5. What year is it?
6. How old are you?
7. What year were you born?
8. What month and day were you born?
9. Who is our president?
10. Who was president before him?

The answer to these questions will quickly give us an idea of the patient's orientation as to time, place, and person. Thus we can guide ourselves as to how to proceed with our rehabilitation program.

Finally, here is a word of caution. I believe we tend to use tranquilizers too freely in stroke patients. While they help to relax the patient, they at the same time make him less responsive to our rehabilitation program, and they may also lower the blood pressure to a point where cerebral blood flow is reduced, when it needs to be maintained for optimum management of the patient. I would therefore prescribe tranquilizers with caution.

PART III
BARRIERS TO STROKE REHABILITATION

Chapter 18

SYSTEMIC BARRIERS

HYPERTENSIVE CARDIOVASCULAR DISEASE
WITH DECOMPENSATION

S INCE the rehabilitation program demands activity, and cardiac decompensation negates strenuous activity, the two are mutually exclusive. Hypertension, per se, however, is not a barrier to rehabilitation. On the contrary, it is often necessary to maintain a certain degree of high blood pressure to overcome the peripheral resistance of the cerebral artherosclerotic vessels. However, if decompensation is present, this must be corrected first, before any strenuous exercise program is undertaken. But to prevent the deleterious effects of inactivity, passive exercise should be prescribed on the ward and should be carried out three times a day, as previously described under "Progressive Rehabilitation— The Bed Phase," Chapter 7. Passive recreational activities on the ward will also help to maintain the patient's morale.

AURICULAR FIBRILLATION

Auricular fibrillation should be corrected before an active program is instituted.

CORONARY INFARCTION

Electrocardiographic examination, which should be done routinely in all C.V.A.'s will often reveal evidence of coronary arteriosclerosis or even evidence of recent or old myocardial infarction. Often such infarction is the cause of the stroke, and may be hidden by it. The objective here is to treat the infarction, which requires prolonged bed rest for the cardiac muscle to heal. Again intensive exercise must be withheld until such healing takes place. The primary objective is to prescribe an exercise program for myocardial infarction. The mainstay of such a program is passive exercise, range of motion of all joints, which is comparable to the early management of a stroke patient. When the cardiologist feels that the patient is ready, then a more active stroke rehabilitation program is instituted.

ANGINA PECTORIS

Effort pain will restrict an active program. However, this can often be controlled by coronary vasodilators, which then will permit the resumption of activity.

URINARY TRACT INFECTION

When associated with fever, urinary tract infection will require appropriate antibiotic management. When the fever subsides, activity can be resumed, and the stroke program can be maintained while the patient is continued on medication.

URINARY INCONTINENCE

Wet, odoriforous clothing is not inviting to the therapist or patient. Rehabilitation activities must await bladder training, which will be discussed later. However, an indwelling or condum catheter which controls such incontinence will permit the patient to continue his stroke routine.

BOWEL INCONTINENCE

Again this is not conducive to patient participation in a stroke rehabilitation program. A bowel training program should be instituted, and if successful, it will permit rehabilitation activities. (See Chapter 21, "Bowel and Bladder Incontinence.)"

SYSTEMIC DISEASES THAT INCAPACITATE AND RESTRICT REHABILITATION EFFORTS

There are some diseases which must be arrested or controlled before rehabilitation can begin. A few are pneumonia, thrombophlebitis, cystitis, bronchial asthma, tuberculosis, and hernia. If symptomatic, such systemic conditions are the first consideration. Only after they have been brought under control can the patient be expected to participate in his stroke rehabilitation activities.

Chapter 19

PHYSICAL BARRIERS TO STROKE REHABILITATION

Tᴴᴇʀᴇ are certain physical problems which render the stroke patient completely or partially resistant to all rehabilitation efforts. These include flexion contractures of the knees, hips, and ankles; knee instability, including genu recurvatum; pain; prolonged flaccidity; edema (hand, wrist, ankle, and foot); and decubiti. We shall now consider them, each in turn.

FLEXION CONTRACTURE OF THE HIPS, KNEES, AND ANKLES

Stroke patients properly cared for from the beginning should not develop flexion contractures, but they do. Where the contracture involves the upper extremity only (Fig. 59), there may be interference with activities of daily living, but of itself, this would not be a contraindication to transfer activities or independent ambulation. But where there is flexion contracture of the hips and knees (Figs. 60, 61), the stroke patient is automatically condemned to a wheelchair existence. For, if the contracture of the hip is more than 150 degrees (0 to 30 degrees based on the anatomical position), the patient's center of gravity is shifted in front of the hip, and he is in trouble even if the knee is straight, because of the accompanying weakness of the paretic lower extremity. If the knee, too, is even partially contracted, ambulation is practically impossible, unless the flexion contractures can be overcome. To do so, Kottke[59] recommends a specific technique which he calls "prolonged counterbalance stretch." While this may be advisable for the younger patients, we have not found it feasible in the older stroke patient. For one thing, it cannot be done without producing pain and discomfort, which the older stroke patient cannot endure. Furthermore, it is questionable whether the potential results are worth the effort. Hence, we

157

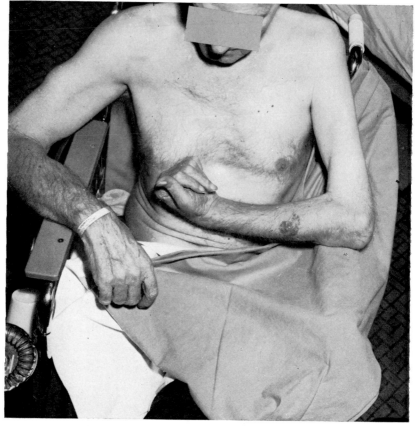

Figure 59. Severe flexion contracture of fingers.

have not attempted this stretching in the older age groups, unless the contracture is recent and minimal. If these patients are able to endure an operation and they give their consent, we prefer surgery. If not, then we have to do the best we can with a permanent independent wheelchair existence.

The sugical treatment for flexion contractures is tenotomy. For plantar flexion contracture of the ankle, we recommend an Achilles tendon tenotomy. For flexion contracture of the knee, the hamstring tendons are partially severed. Iliopsoas tenotomy can be performed for severe hip flexion contracture. If successful, such operations may help to convert a wheelchair patient to at

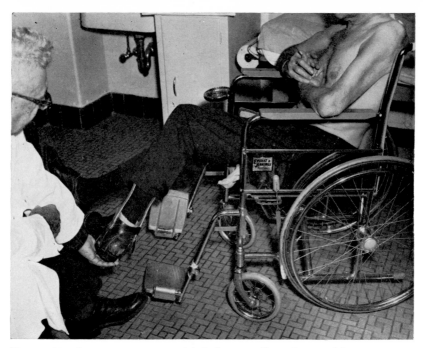

Figure 60. Flexion contracture of left fingers, elbow, hip, and knee. Patient is restricted to a wheelchair existence.

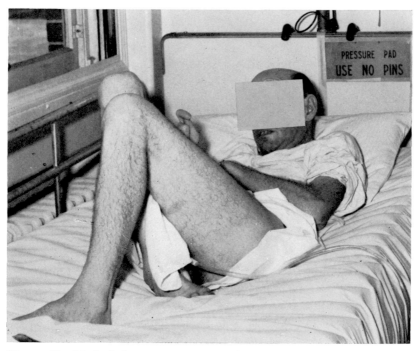

Figure 61. Marked flexion contracture of nonparetic, and paretic lower extremities, as well as both wrists and fingers. Patient is completely helpless.

least a partially ambulatory state. Again, it must be emphasized that the best treatment for contractures is prevention. Exercise, exercise, and more exercise, passive, active assistive, and if possible, active, from the beginning, will help prevent this obstacle to rehabilitation.

UNSTABLE KNEE

Ambulation requires a stable knee. In younger patients, building up the quadriceps by progressive resistance exercises will overcome the cruciate or collateral ligament instability and thus help to maintain stability of the knee. In the older stroke patients, such exercise is not possible or feasible. Hence, the only way possible for these patients to walk is to supply them with a knee cage or long leg brace (Fig. 23 a and b).

PAIN

Fortunately, pain is not a common symptom in stroke patients. When it occurs with associated conditions, such as arthritis, these become the indication for treatment. But pain does occur and is of two types: (a) thalamic pain, and (b) shoulder-hand syndrome. *Thalamic* pain has already been discussed under "Dysesthesia" (See Chapter 15). This pain will not as a rule interfere with stroke rehabilitation. It will require some type of tranquilizer. It will usually gradually disappear. The shoulder-hand syndrome is another matter. It manifests itself by pain in the shoulder, usually in the acromioclavicular region and radiates down to the arm and fingers. It is due to immobility, which in turn results in deltoid atrophy. It is aggravated by failure to support the arm by a shoulder sling. Examination of such patients will often reveal a space between the acromion process of the scapula and the tuberosity of the humerus.

Treatment is as follows: For pain relief, the usual physical therapy modalities are indicated, namely a hot pack to the shoulder followed by effleurage. A shoulder sling should be provided for the patient to wear (Fig. 89 a and b) if he is ambulatory, or a wheelchair rest when he is in the wheelchair (Figs. 54 to 57). Stimulation of the deltoid can be tried with a sinusoidal or dynawave current in an attempt to improve deltoid strength. Analgesics will also help to encourage the patient to continue with his program.

PROLONGED FLACCIDITY

In the majority of patients, after a short interval of flaccid paralysis following the C.V.A., spasticity sets in and gradually increases in the paralyzed upper and lower extremities. The management of spasticity has been discussed in Chapter 14. Occasionally, however, the flaccid paralysis persists and becomes a definite hindrance to a good rehabilitation routine, unless corrective steps are taken. A trial of ambulation with a short or long leg brace will be required to permit the patient to walk, and probably a crutch or cane will be necessary. As already indicated concerning the shoulder-hand syndrome, where the upper extremity is flaccid, a shoulder sling during walking, and/or a pad on the wheelchair for the paretic arm when sitting, and stimulation of the deltoid may help prevent the shoulder-hand syndrome, and permit the patient to continue with his program. This support of the paretic arm is necessary for a second reason, namely to prevent swelling of the hand and wrist because of the slowing of the venous return from the distal part of the extremity, caused by dependence.

EDEMA OF THE HAND, WRIST, ANKLE, AND FOOT

The cause of edema of the hand and wrist and, sometimes, forearm is dependency, with its slowing of the venous return. The prevention is a sling suspension of the shoulder when the patient is walking and an arm rest on the wheelchair when he is sitting. The treatment for the swelling, if moderate, is centripetal massage. If, however, the swelling is fairly marked, the best treatment is intermittent mechanical compression produced by one of the compression units now available. For stasis swelling of the foot, ankle, and leg, apply centripetal massage or intermittent mechanical compresson, followed by a properly fitting elastic stocking.

DECUBITI

Malleolar decubitus should not be an obstacle to rehabilitation.

If the patient is able to walk, he should be permitted to continue to walk, and the decubitus will heal fairly rapidly with the help of local ultraviolet, five seconds at contact, daily. We have also had good results with small decubiti by the employment of a sinusoidal or a dynawave current over the decubitus, five minutes daily to toleration (Figs. 62-64). A large or infected decubitus over the malleolus, or heel, is a definite obstacle to walking and requires more prolonged care, including daily dressing with an antibiotic ointment, such as neosporin.® These take a long time to heal. The patient should not be permited to bear weight until the infection has subsided. To prevent such decubiti in the ankle, cover it with self-adhering material made from polyether urethane foam.⁶⁰

Sacral or ischial decubiti are a definite barrier to stroke re-

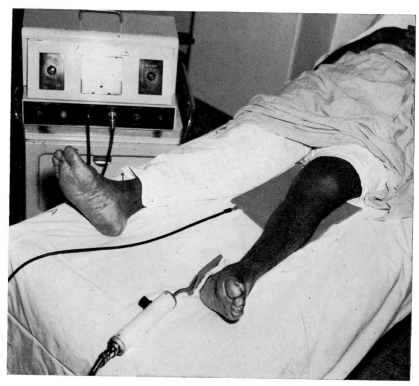

Figure 62. Application of Dynawave current.

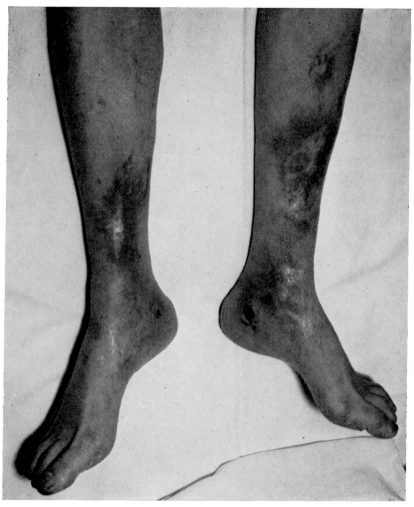

Figure 63. Small decubitus on medial malleolus.

habilitation. Once they have been allowed to develop, and I say allowed, because in most cases proper care of the patient, including frequent turning, will prevent such complications, they are very difficult to heal. But they can heal in time if appropriate measures are taken. These include, for example, a Royalaire air-fluidized bed (Milton Roy Company, P.O. Box 1219, St. Petersburg, Florida, 33733), or Hydro-float Flotation Pad for Bed or

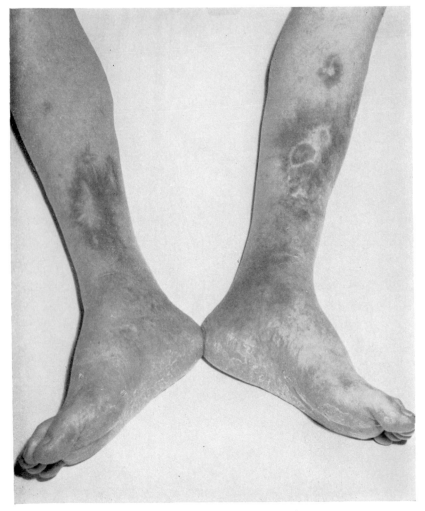

Figure 64. Same area after a month's treatment with Dynawave current.

Wheelchair (Jobst Institute Inc., Box 653, Toledo, Ohio, 43601), or Ortho Decubiti Pillow for bed or wheelchair (Ortho Industries, Inc., 49 Lawton St., New Rochelle, New York, 10801).

Weinstein and Davidson noted a markedly diminished pressure, by at least two thirds, over the usual pressure areas, produced by a fluid-support mattress and seat.[61]

Chapter 20

MENTAL BARRIERS TO STROKE REHABILITATION

W HILE systemic or physical barriers to stroke rehabilitation are generally obvious and are easily detected, this is not true of mental barriers. These usually are hidden, and often the members of the stroke rehabilitation team, unless looking for them, will not recognize them and will accuse the patient of "lack of motivation." We hear such expressions as the patient "won't cooperate," or "he just doesn't want to help himself," or "the patient is not motivated." Sometimes even the physician is unaware of the underlying mental condition and will reprimand the patient for his noncooperation. It is possible, of course, that some patients have a good potential for rehabilitation, but are motivated the wrong way, that is, *not to get better,* either for social gain or monetary compensation. These, for the most part, are recognized for what they are, and efforts to help them are wasted as long as it pays them to stay handicapped. And there are others with a severe degree of cerebral encephalopathy, again recognizable, whose mental capacity for rehabilitation is nil. They will remain dependent patients except, perhaps, that they may be amenable to certain minimal self-care activities, such as feeding themselves.

But there is a third group of patients whose rehabilitation potential is restricted by mental barriers which will not be recognized, unless suspected and looked for. Hence, if a patient seems to be resistant to activity, we have to try to determine why, and if possible, help him overcome his resistance.

To evaluate these mental barriers, the first step is to determine whether the patient's stroke is the cause of his problem or whether the problem anteceded the stroke. This determination is made by obtaining a history from his family, from his physician, and from previous hospitalizations, if any.

165

PAST HISTORY OF MENTAL DIFFICULTY

Specifically, the rehabilitation team wants to know the following: (1) What kind of a person are we dealing with? (a) Has he always been high-strung, irritable, easy to react to slight provocation? (b) Is there a history of anxiety? Has he been annoyed by little things? (c) Is there a history of moodiness? Changing from elation to depression, from laughter to tears, from joy to sorrow? (d) Is there a history of dependency? Has the patient been inclined to lean on his mother, as a youth, or his older sisters or brothers, or some friend, or since marriage, has he been dependent on his spouse, and has not made independent decisions, always letting someone else decide for him? (e) Has he been known to have a chip on his shoulder? Has he been negative, hostile, antagonistic? (f) Is there a history of phobias, particularly fear of illness, fear of death? (g) Is there a history of denial of illness? This does not mean, as is true with some people, that they make light of their troubles, just as others exaggerate them. It means, for example, that a person has an obvious physical defect, such as a swollen ankle, and he says, "No, the ankle is not swollen, I wore the wrong shoes this morning." (h) Is there a history of a "nervous breakdown." Find out if this was another name for an acute psychosis or severe psychoneurosis. How was it treated? What was his response to treatment? With such background, a person suffering from a stroke may be expected to show an intensification of his previous symptoms, rather than an alleviation.

PAST HISTORY NONCONTRIBUTORY

Let us assume that the patient has a negative or noncontributory past history of mental difficulty. He was a good average citizen, a good son, a good student, a good husband, a good father, a good provider or homemaker, a steady, well-rounded individual. He has had a stroke, and now he is an obvious management problem. In view of this, is it fair to assume that he just will not cooperate or that he is not motivated? Before we come to such a decision, we must assess (a) the type of brain damage, (b) its localization, and (c) the extent of brain involvement. The neurologist or neurosurgeon has already helped us with the answer to these questions. Now, it is necessary to determine the psychological effect of this damage. The answer then is a psychological evaluation. Many tests have been developed to determine the effect of brain damage upon an individual and his response thereto. Allison[62] tested patients from the standpoint of appearance, mood, level of consciousness, speech, behavior, memory, intellect, and body awareness.

Adams and Hurwitz[63] used a square pegboard with pegs grouped distinctly at four corners with which to test the patient's ability to locate the pegs in the right spots. They studied forty-five stroke patients who could not be taught self-care and ambulation, and analyzed their subjects from the following standpoints: level of consciousness, speech impairment, behavioral difficulties, memory, intellectual impairment, and body awareness.

They found the following reasons for their patient's invalidism: (a) severe motor, sensory, and mental defects; (b) marked obesity and its accompanying indolence; (c) occipital blindness; (d) other disturbances, such as amputation, eye difficulties, and respiratory affections; (e) poor comprehension; (f) lost body awareness, manifested by neglect or denial; (g) apraxic gait pattern, i.e. difficulty with continued walking; (h) marked postural imbalance; and (i) those just unwilling to cooperate.

Bruel and Peszczynski[64] have shown that hemiplegic patients have a disturbed perception of verticality, namely they see vertical objects as if they were in an inclined position. Birch *et al.*[65] found that the stroke patients had disturbed perception in both vertical and horizontal spheres. Birch *et al.*, studying visual verticality in hemiplegia,[66] noted that the deficit of hemiplegic patients seemed to be an inability of the nervous system to bring the five senses into close touch with one another, rather than a lack of any of the senses.

The point I wish to make is that the members of the rehabilitation team should try to recognize these underlying aberrations and discuss them at the team meetings, so that the physician may then ask for psychological evaluation and psychiatric help in the possible hope of overcoming some of these barriers to rehabilitation. What then should the team members look for?

GUIDELINES TO LOOKING FOR OBSTACLES
TO REHABILITATION

1. Ask the patient to stand up. He cannot maintain the correct posture even with his eyes open. Ask him to sit up. He still cannot do it. Now ask him to try the same with his eyes closed. He is much worse. Obviously he is suffering from some type of dysequilibrium. Tell the patient what you mean by correct sitting or standing, point it out to him, and show him by your example just what you mean. He still cannot sit or stand upright. We say that he has lost the ability to maintain the correct posture. The question is why? (a) He cannot physically do it. (b) He is mentally ill. (c) He does not want to do it. A psychological evaluation will help determine which it is.

2. Now ask the patient to move his limbs in bed. He does so without difficulty, and takes all his joints through complete range of motion. Now ask him to stand up and walk. He cannot move his limbs at all. The problem is *apraxia of motion*. The treatment here is to try bicycle exercises or rowing, with the hope that this can be overcome.

3. Place a spoon in front of the patient; ask the patient to put the spoon in his mouth. He does not recognize the spoon. Try, "Pour water from the pitcher into the glass." He does not recognize the objects. This is *visual or auditory agnosia*. The speech pathologist will be helpful here at least to label the difficulty.

4. Ask the patient to move his paretic arm. He moves it, full range, but says "I can't do it." I asked one patient, who, in response to the request, moved his arm and at the same time said "I can't do it." I said, "What are you moving? Isn't this your arm?" He said, "No, this is my brother's arm." This is denial of illness or *anosognosia*. A common example of anosognosia is the almost invariable tendency of a stroke patient to cover his paretic arm.

5. Ask the patient to raise his nonparetic hand. He does so. Ask him to close his eyes. He again raises his hand. This is *perseveration*.

6. Ask the patient to look at you and keep on looking. He looks at you and immediately takes his eyes away from you. This is *impersistence*.

7. Ask him to open a book or pick up a pencil. Now say to him "What did I ask you to do?" He does not remember. This is *loss of memory for recent events.*

8. Show him a photo of a person, someone in the day's newspaper. Ask him to point to the person's nose or eyes. He cannot do it. Then you point to the nose or eyes, and ask him to name them. He does so accurately. This is called *disturbance of body image.*

9. Ask him to move the right hand forward. He moves both hands forward. This is a form of *dyskinesia.*

10. Ask him to pick up a penny or a dime. He says, "I don't want to do it." This could be a form of *depression.*

11. Ask him to write his name. He does so. You say, "That's fine, you're doing well," and he starts crying. Or tell him "You look fine," and he starts crying. This is *thalamic crying.* Or he will start laughing or crying for no apparent reason.

12. Put a chair in the center of the room. Ask him to walk by it. He bumps into it. This is *space blindness.*

SUMMARY

It is necessary for the rehabilitation team to recognize the deficiencies and to ask for appropriate help to overcome them if possible. They may endanger the patient's health, and even life. They certainly are an obstacle to rehabilitation. Caution the family and the institutional personnel, if he is institutionalized, that he should not be left alone. He may light a match and forget to put it out, or he may put a pot of water on the stove and forget about it and let it boil over, or he may bump into objects and hurt himself, or he may fall and break his hip.

On the other hand, it must not be forgotten that, whatever their deficiencies, these are human beings with feelings like those of other human beings. We should, therefore, arrange our rehabilitation program to suit them, not us. Or, we may ask them to do something which they cannot do, for one reason or another, and thus hinder rather than help them to attain their goal.

And finally a word about "motivation." Let us say that we have carefully reviewed all the possible barriers to the patient's rehabilitation and apparently did not find any; yet the patient still does not respond to our efforts. A careful study by Belmont,[67] comparing stroke patients and other handicapped patients, but without brain damage, has indicated that therapist-patient interaction resulted in increased patient participation for the stroke patients but not for those without brain damage. I have found this true in general, and specifically in the S.A.E. routine, where the degree of improvement has varied considerably with the therapist's, or therapy aide's, or even family's presence and encouragement. The average stroke patient does not have the mental capacity to go it alone. And when I refer to the therapist's presence and participation, I mean participation in his activity and not a discussion of extraneous subjects.

Chapter 21

BOWEL AND BLADDER INCONTINENCE

W E have considered barriers to stroke rehabilitation under three headings, systemic, physical, and mental. We now come to a type of barrier which encompasses all three, namely bowel and bladder incontinence. As already indicated, it is difficult, if not impossible, to undertake a satisfactory rehabilitation program as long as there is a bowel or bladder incontinence. It is utterly unfair to expect a therapist to work with such a patient. It is unfair to the patient himself, to expect him to participate in any activity while he, his clothes, and his surroundings are soiled with malodorous urine or feces. It is, therefore, necessary to attempt to overcome this objectionable situation by a program of bowel and bladder training which we shall now discuss.

BOWEL AND BLADDER TRAINING PROGRAM

Principles

In order for a patient to be trained in satisfactory bowel and bladder function, he must be fairly well oriented. A mentally incompetent patient will not respond to any training program. Such a patient will have to be satisfied with appropriate bowel and bladder care, i.e. routine enemas and catheterizations. Where feasible, external catheter drainage is much preferable to a constant indwelling catheter.

A schedule for defecation and urination should be established and maintained. This schedule should be consistent with the patient's prestroke pattern, where such is known. This means that if a patient has been in the habit of having a regular bowel movement on arising, training should take cognizance of this habit. Or if he has had frequency of urination and nocturia before his stroke, as, for example, the result of a benign prostatic hypertrophy, this too has to be considered in his bladder-training program.

171

Prerequisites

The first and most important prerequisite is the patient's cooperation. This means that the patient will respond to the direction of the nursing staff. This is why we said that he must be mentally competent. A mentally incompetent patient is not suitable for such a program.

The second prerequisite is that the program be organized, both as to plan and execution.

The Program

The program involves the patient, the nurse, and the plan itself.

I. The patient

1. Remember that he is a person, has a name, and family, and is a member of society. He has feelings and emotions just like you and me. He is not happy with his incontinence and wants to help overcome it.
2. Even if the patient is dysphasic, do not assume that he is necessarily disoriented. On the contrary act on the basis that he is aware of his environment.
3. Encourage the patient to keep trying and commend him for even a slight accomplishment.
4. If necessary, use diapers in the beginning, but discard them as soon as feasible.
5. Remove the indwelling catheter. If necessary to empty the bladder, reinsert the catheter. But try not to keep catheter in the bladder for any length of time. This is how cystitis develops with its complications of ureteritis and pyelonephritis.
6. Avoid frequent enemas. They irritate the rectum and cause atony of the colon.

II. The nursing staff

1. Establish rapport with the patient. Encourage friendly relations and mutual understanding.
2. Consult with the physician and with patient's family.
3. Establish proper liaison with the other members of the team. Explain what you are doing. Ask them to report their observations.

4. Study bowel and bladder evacuation. Have your team-mates observe and report to you. Observe frequency, type, amount, color, consistency, and odor. If indicated, have feces and urine examined by laboratory. It is generally accepted by progressive physicians in charge of rehabilitation that a trained nurse can and should palpate the abdomen, and even do a rectal for possible detection of fecal impaction, and possible manual removal of such inspissated feces.

5. Keep in touch with the doctor and the other members of the team concerning the patient's progress in other areas.

III. The training program

  A. General rules for bowel and bladder retraining

Force fluids. Check urine reaction, try to maintain an acid urine, by proper diet and medication, if needed. The diet should be acid ash, should include cranberry juice, and should limit orange and lemon juice, and milk. If the urine is cloudy and alkaline and the doctor approves, the patient may be given ammonium chloride tablets (0.5 gm), three times a day, until the urine is clear.

Have patient turned in bed, at least every two hours. Provide him with a trapeze bar and encourage him to use it. Give passive exercises to paretic limbs and encourage active exercises for nonparetic limbs. Do this as often as possible, but at least three times a day. Teach the patient to use nonparetic limbs with which to move the paretic limbs. Get the patient out of bed into a wheelchair as soon as his condition warrants. As soon as feasible, start ambulation training, first between parallel bars, then outside of bars, using any assists available. Continue exercises. Avoid the use of a bed pan. Have the patient sit on a commode chair or better still, on a toilet seat. Teach him the proper semisquat position.

  B. Specific directions for bowel retraining

    1. For a responsive patient

      a. As already indicated, check with doctor, family, and with patient himself as to previous bowel habits.

b. Palpate abdomen for any lumpiness.

c. Insert gloved finger in rectum to note any fecal impaction.

d. If impaction is noted, then administer olive oil enema.

e. In the morning, insert DuLcolax® suppository as far as you can reach.

f. Give patient breakfast meal.

g. Have patient hold suppository, thirty minutes, if possible. The object of DuLcolax suppository is to stimulate colon contraction. The breakfast meal acts similarly.)

h. As patient shows improvement, change from DuLcolax to glycerin suppository.

i. Eliminate suppository and encourage spontaneous evacuation.

j. Continue to serve breakfast, including fruit juices, at regular hours, and have patient attempt bowel evacuation at routine time.

k. If necessary repeat suppository before lunch.

2. Bowel care for nonresponsive patient

a. Insert suppository, as above.

b. Wait thirty minutes and place on bed pan.

C. Specific directions for bladder retraining

1. For responsive patient

a. Observe frequency and time of urination.

b. Measure intake and output.

c. Place patient on commode, if possible, or bed pan, if necessary, every two hours while awake and every three hours at night. For male patients, offer urinal, and instruct him to sit up in bed with feet hanging over edge of bed, to use urinal.

d. Note patient's timing of urination, i.e. record his voiding schedule.

e. The next day, place patient on bed pan, or offer him urinal, consistent with his previously noted voiding schedule.

f. If he continues to wet the bed, place on bed pan, or give urinal, fifteen minutes before expected wetting time, and keep him on pan fifteen minutes.

   g. If necessary, stimulate with cold water to bladder or by pressure on bladder.

2. For incontinent male

Put condum catheter around penis and proceed as above. Precaution: do not compress penis too tightly.

3. For incontinent female

Use abdominal pad covered by plastic and held in place by sanitary belt, and proceed as above.

Note: Pending the restoration of bowel and bladder continence, it is often advisable to eliminate the offensive odors perfusing the atmosphere. A Derifil® tablet administered to such patient daily will often make the difference between an acceptable and a malolorous ward.

Chapter 22

SPECIAL PROBLEMS

W E shall now consider two special problems in connection with stroke rehabilitation. The first is accidental, and the second, even more important, is incidental. I am referring to fractured hip, and above-the-knee amputations in stroke patients.

FRACTURE OF THE HIP

More correctly this should be called fracture of the neck of the femur. As already indicated in the past chapters, we are dealing here with older patients, who bones are osteoporotic and, therefore, brittle. It does not take much of a fall to produce a fracture, usually of the neck of the femur of the paretic lower extremity. A fall out of bed or a fall while attempting to walk without supervision will often result in this complication. X-rays will confirm such fracture, and the patient then becomes a special management problem.

Management of Fracture of the Hip

If the patient is amenable to surgical interference, and gives his consent therefor, an open reduction with hip fixation will permit resumption of activity as soon as the postoperative condition warrants. For most patients, however, operation is not feasible, and a serious question arises as to management. The older people cannot be treated like young hip fracture patients with open reduction, hip fixation, casting, and prolonged immobilization. The best routine for these patients is to get them out of bed, provide them with a pair of crutches, and teach them to use them with minimal weight bearing on the fractured lower extremity. If the paretic arm is too weak to permit crutch ambulation, then they should at least be wheeled to the parallel bars or given a walker, and allowed to stand on the nonparetic leg a few minutes every hour, again with minimal weight bearing on the fractured

176

limb. Meanwhile, the rest of the rehabilitation program proceeds without too much interruption, i.e. exercise to the nonparetic upper and lower extremities and the paretic upper extremity, self-care, occupational therapy and speech therapy, where indicated.

ABOVE THE KNEE AMPUTATIONS

Many of the stroke patients have diabetes and arteriosclerosis obliterans. It is not surprising, therefore, that so many develop arteriosclerotic and/or diabetic gangrene requiring amputation. An amputation below the knee is serious, but not as difficult in terms of rehabilitation as one above the knee. Here we are starting with a paresis on one side of the body, and weakness of the other side, perhaps dysphasia, dysesthesia, and dysmentia. The superimposition of an above the knee amputation would seem to make the task of rehabilitation impossible. Yet, we have had innumerable patients who have had such amputations and have made a good rehabilitation adjustment. Where the patient's condition permits, we frequently supply him with an artificial limb and train him in its use. When the patient is obviously unable to manipulate such a prosthesis, because of general weakness, weak heart, or inadequate strength in the nonparetic lower extremity, or where the paretic upper extremity is functionless, the prescription of a prosthesis is usually contraindicated. To manipulate an above-knee prosthesis requires a great deal of energy and training. Of course, if the patient can afford it or he is a veteran with a potential for survival for more than six months, we sometimes supply him with a limb for cosmetic and social purposes, like going to church. But we make clear to the patient that he will wear the limb, but not be able to walk with it.

The routine for a stroke patient with an above-the-knee amputation is to prepare the stump for a prosthesis, by preprosthetic training and stump conditioning, including massage and wrapping. Where there is a stump neuroma, we treat that with ultrasound, usually one watt per square centimeter, five minutes daily. When the stump and patient are ready, we measure him for a prosthesis and order the same from the prosthetist. While the limb is being made, we continue to give him stump conditioning and preprosthetic training, consisting of walking on one leg between parallel bars, followed, if feasible, by crutch ambulation, first inside, then outside the bars.

The usual prescription for an above-knee amputation prosthesis is as follows: Conventional A. K. prosthesis with a SACH molded foot, wood laminated shank, quadrilateral socket, Bock safety knee, pelvic belt suspension with hip control, and three three-ply and three five-ply socks.

This is varied sometimes to give the elderly patient a shoulder harness. For the patient who has a slight flexion contracture of the hip, we prescribe a standarfd wood foot, instead of a SACH foot, so as to permit the patient to place his entire foot on the ground during the stance phase of ambulation, something which the SACH foot does not permit under such circumstances.

When the limb arrives and the patient is properly fitted, we institute prosthetic training, first between parallel bars, then with crutches between bars, then crutches outside bars, on level ground, up and down steps, up and down a ramp, until we feel that the patient is able to handle his prosthesis satisfactorily. For the younger and stronger patient we try ambulation with a cane, to see if this is feasible. The older patient, however, usually is satisfied with crutch ambulation. Often, we also supply him with a wheelchair for home use so that he does not have to go to the trouble of putting on his prosthesis every time he wants to negotiate a short distance, as going from bed to toilet.

A few examples will help to illustrate some of the problems of above the knee amputations in stroke patients.

Case 1

A.M., fifty-five, C.V.A., 1962, right hemiplegia, and dysphasia, on Dilantin® for seizures, fair recovery as to ambulation, poor recovery as to speech, minimal motion in upper extremity. September 27, 1966, right A.K. amputation for A.S.O. Patient had a prolonged convalescence.

As we were not sure of patient's ability to walk with a prosthesis, we ordered a temporary prothesis, which was made at our own brace shop. Patient seemed to be able to handle this, so on April 7, 1967 we ordered a permanent prosthesis with wood foot, as outlined above. Figure 65 a, b, c, May 3, 1967, shows

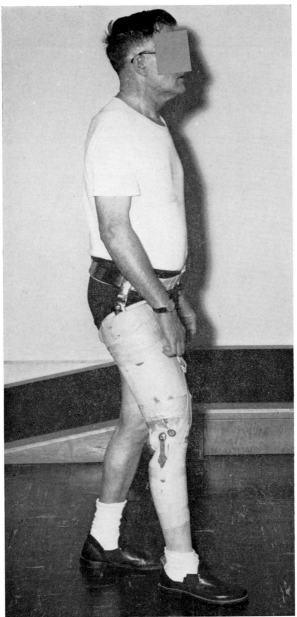

Figure 65. a. *(this page)*, b., and c.—(A.M.) Old right hemiplegia; areriosclerosis obliterans; right A. K. amputation (4-7-67). (5-3-67) patient walking with unfinished prosthesis.

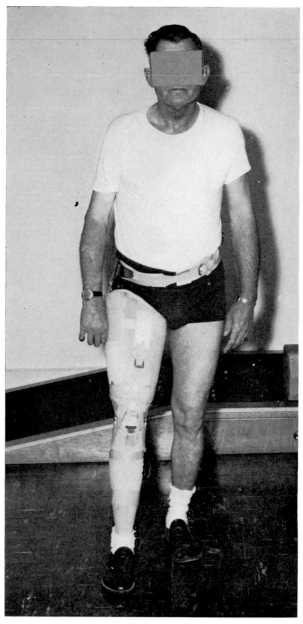

Figure 65b.

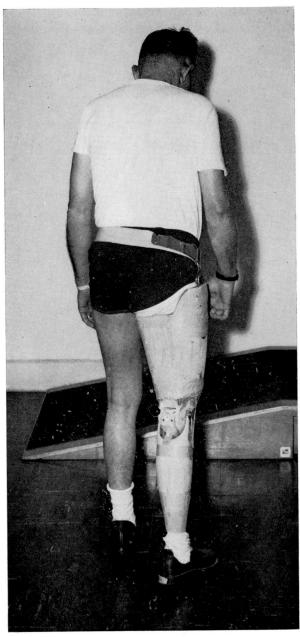

Figure 65c.

patient walking with unfinished limb. Patient was discharged on May 30, 1967, able to walk with or without cane.

Case 2

J.L.E., fifty-six, C.V.A. 1962, discharged with good motion both upper and left lower extremities, minimal motion right lower extremity. Readmitted, April 9, 1969 because of ulcer right leg. Oscillographic studies showed diminished pulsations both lower extremities consistent with A.S.O. October 23, 1969, right A.K. amputation; December 17, 1969, we ordered a right A.K. prosthesis, as above outlined, with pelvic belt and single shoulder strap suspension. March 18, 1970, patient discharged with crutches. (Fig. 66 a, b, c.)

Case 3

D.A.R, seventy-six, old left hemiplegia. Left A.K. amputation. Because of age and general weakness, patient was supplied with a wheelchair, as not being suitable for prosthesis (Fig. 67).

Case 4

C.D.P., fifty-two, textile worker. C.V.A., 1959, right hemiplegia, mild dysphasia; returned to work. April 17, 1970, right A.K. amputation for gangrene right foot. Oscillographic studies showed diminished pulsations left lower extremity. We ordered a standard A.K. prosthesis first with SACH, then with wood foot. Figure 68 a, b, shows patient walking with prosthesis between parallel bars. Figure 68 c, d, patient walking outside bars with SACH foot. Figure 68e, patient walking with wood foot.

Note: When ordering a wheelchair for a stroke amputee, be sure it is a special *amputee wheelchair,* in which the rear wheels are set back to compensate for the loss of limb. Also specify "removable arms," to permit the patient to get into and out of the chair more easily.

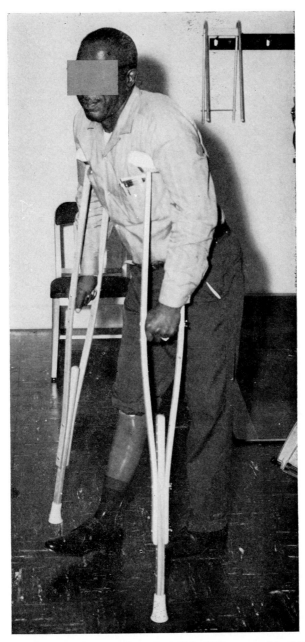

Figure 66. a. *(this page)*, b., and c.—(J.L.E.) (56) years-old, C.V.A., 1962.
Right A. K. amputation (October 23, 1969) for arteriosclerosis obliterans;
prolonged convalescence.

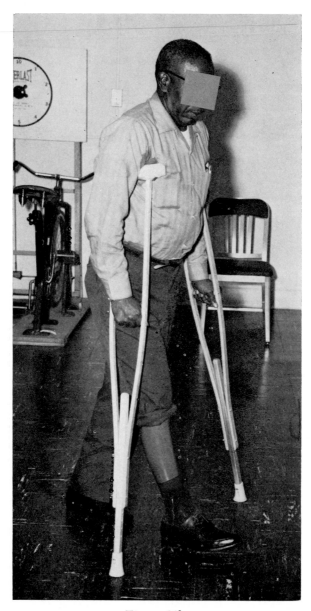

Figure 66b.

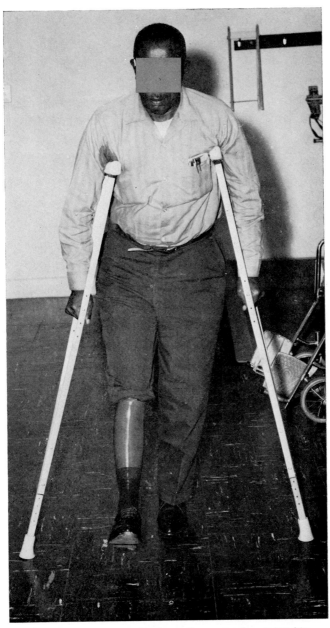

Figure 66c. Patient discharged on crutches 3/18/70

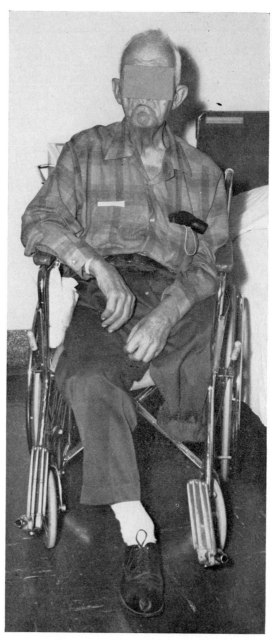

Figure 67. (D.A.R.) Seventy-six years old. Left hemiplegia (October 23, 1969). Rt. A.K. amputation. Patient not suitable for prosthesis, issued wheelchair.

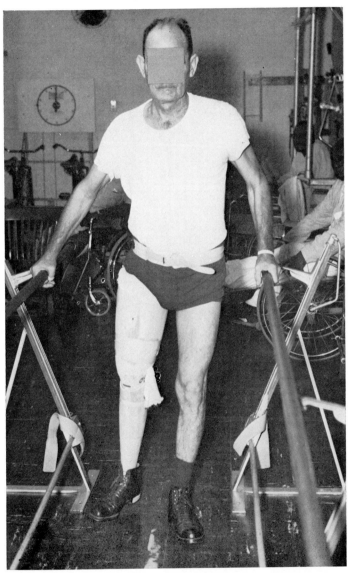

Figure 68. (C.D.P.) Fifty-two years old, textile worker (1959), (Right hemiplegia, mild dysphasia) returned to work. (4-17-70) Right A.K. amputation for gangrene right foot; Figure 68a. *(this page)* and b.—patient walking with unfinished right A.K. prosthesis between parallel bars.

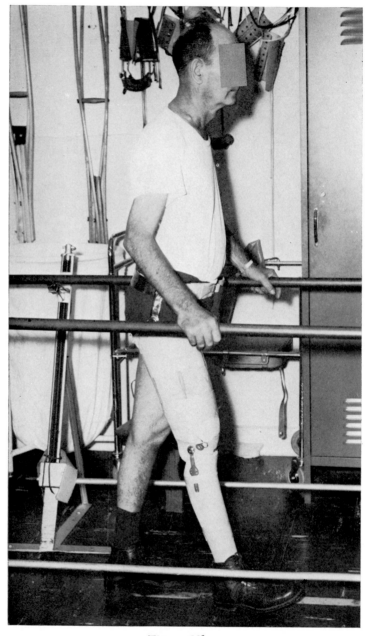

Figure 68b.

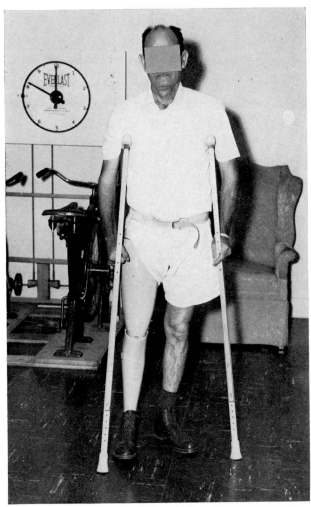

Figure 68c. Figure 68c and d—Walking with finished right A.K. prosthesis and SACH foot, and two crutches.

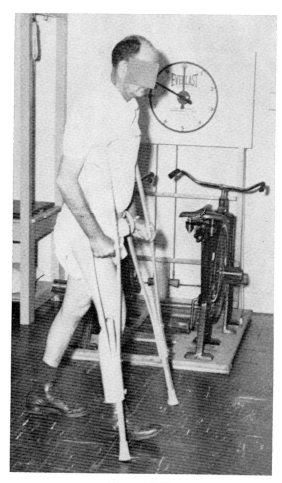

Figure 68d.

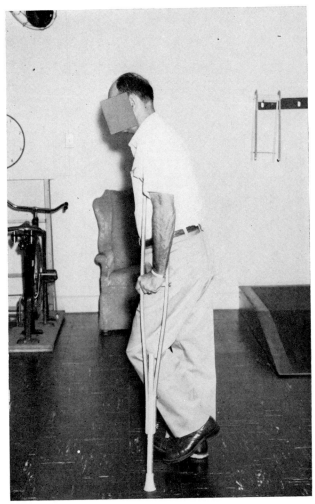

Figure 68e. Walking with right A.K. prosthesis and wood foot, which now can be placed flat on ground.

PART IV
ACTIVITIES OF DAILY LIVING

Chapter 23

A.D.L.–ACTIVITIES OF DAILY LIVING

INTRODUCTION

I N previous chapters we have discussed the general considerations of stroke rehabilitation, the stroke 4-dys-syndrome, the barriers to stroke rehabilitations, and special problems. We now come to the part in our manual which may seem rather prosaic; but to the stroke patient with residual disability, it is just as important as the actual rehabilitation program. In this chapter we shall discuss the procedures which make the difference between a satisfactory, self-dependent existence or a state of dependency. Hence, this section may be called *a program for self-care*. While it is true that some members of society thrive on being waited on, most of us prefer to do things for ourselves. Therefore, it is up to the members of the rehabilitation team to assist the stroke patient to develop as much potential for self-care as his residual condition warrants. This is why we provide these patients with certain assistive devices, so as to permit them to do the possible. But we should not ask them to attempt the unreasonable. I have emphasized again and again that these recovered or, if you will, rehabilitated patients are not physiologically normal. They still have the potential for a second or a third or even a fourth stroke, so we must make life for them not difficult, but reasonably easy; not strenuous and complicated, but unstrained and simple.

To help these people to live, and if possible to enjoy life, a number of assistive devices have already been developed, and more are being constantly produced. In the following pages, I shall present some of the most commonly used assists and indicate how they are used. For a more complete listing of such devices, the reader is referred to the various bulletins and catalogues which will be found at the end of the book (Appendix B).

MOBILITY ASSISTS

In Chapter 8, we discussed wheelchairs. We mentioned the standard metal wheelchair. This is the most useful and practical, but there are other chairs that may be used. Some of these will now be considered.

The Hemichair

This chair (Fig. 69, Everest and Jennings) has all the advantages of the standard chair plus the additional feature of being more suitable for maneuvering with one hand and one foot. This is made possible by placing all the controls both for movement and braking on the nonparetic side of the patient. Not all patients, however, are able to use this chair, since it requires a greater

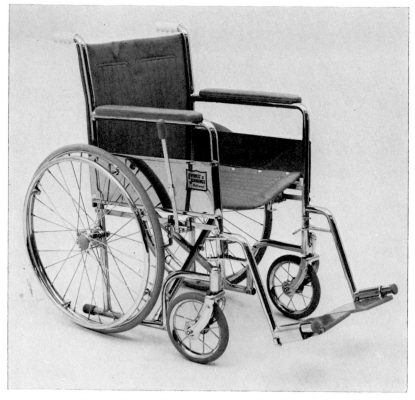

Figure 69. a. *(this page)* and b.—The hemichair.

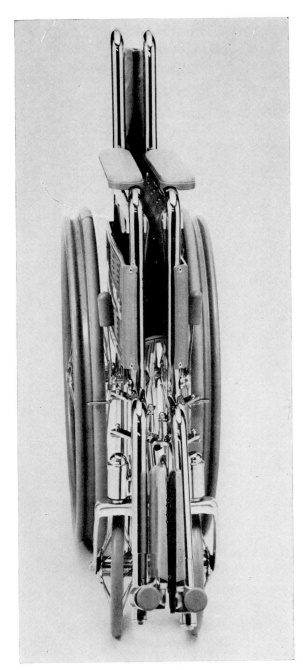

Figure 69b.

effort of concentration than the standard chair. But for those whose mental status permits its use, it is a definite advantage over the regular wheel chair.

Power Drive Chair

For the patient with poor cardiac reserve or poor respiratory reserve, a power chair is available with push-knob control and speed selector. The chair can be folded.

Monodrive Chair

The monodrive chair or monodrive attachments for a standard wheelchair are available with left-hand or right-hand controls. The latter can be attached to a standard chair and can be raised out of the way when so desired by the patient. If a permanent attachment is desired, this too can be provided. Electric chairs are now equipped with a battery and a battery charger which permits six to eight hours of power between charges.

Note: Before an individual purchases a wheelchair, he should consult with his physician as to the best type for his specific needs.

WALKING ASSISTS

For those patients who are unable to use a standard cane or crutch, walking aids are available ranging from Quad canes with four point ground contact (Everest and Jennings), or Rehab canes (Shalik), to Tripod canes (Cleo), to standard walkers, or rolling aids (walkers with casters). The walkers are of two types: (a) folding, open end, or closed end, and (b) non-folding. For additional support, they may be ordered with crutch attachments or balance ring attachments. An additional walker is available that can be controlled with either hand for those patients who have no function at all in the paretic upper extremity. This is a one-handed walker (Shalik). It has the standard four legs plus an additional fifth leg in front with an extension for grasping with one hand, either hand. For walkers with casters, a hand brake is available (Invalex).

Utilization of Walking Assists

All walking assists represent an added support to the body to supplement the diminished support by the paretic leg. The type of assist, therefore, will depend on the residual strength of the paretic leg. The stronger the paretic leg, the less support needed; the weaker the paretic leg, the more support needed. While the professional members of the team can suggest the type of assist needed, ultimately the patient himself and his immediate family will be the final judges of the best support for his individual needs. All must remember, however, that safety precautions should always be stressed. Crutches, canes, and walkers should be equipped with rubber, nonskid safety tips. There should be no loose scattered rugs upon which the patient can trip. The carpeting in the house should be skid-proof. The patient should be reminded always to keep the walking assist near him and never, never to take any chances of taking even a single step without it.

A fifty-three-year-old man with a residual weakness of right lower extremity perfectly able to walk with one crutch, was watching television, got up to change the station, forgot about his crutch, fell, and sustained an intertrochanteric fracture of his right femur. The hip had to be pinned, and the patient was unable to resume his walking for six months.

SELF-FEEDING AIDS

The stroke patient with one functional hand will need equipment that will permit him to feed himself with only one hand, although the patient should be encouraged to use the other paretic hand as an assist. What he will need, therefore, is a dish to keep the food from falling off, as he scoops it out; a combination knife and fork with which to cut and lift the food to his mouth; a rocker knife for cutting his meat with one hand; also a combination of spoon and fork. Some of these will be described. Additional aids can be obtained from various catalogs to be listed at the end of the book. To keep the solid food from falling off the plate, as it is scooped out, one can use a food guard attachment to the regular plate. The simplest food guard clamps on the plate by spring action. Other food guards use a rubber fastener for attachment to the plate. The advantage of this is that the rubber between plate and table prevents the plate from sliding. However, another way to prevent the plate from sliding is the use of a suction plate in which three suction cups are placed at the outer edge of the plate and pressed to the table top.

The meat-cutter knife has a large wooden or plastic or ivory-like handle and a long curved blade.

The knife and fork combination has a similar handle to the rocking knife except that the end of the knife is serrated into a fork like appearance.

TOILET AIDS

The most important aids for self-care toilet activities are (a) the installation of proper support bars, and (b) the adjustment of the toilet to the proper height of the patient.

The support bar is needed to help the patient to sit down on and stand up from the toilet seat. The bar may be a handrail at 45 degrees fastened to the wall, or a right angle rail fastened to the wall and floor, or one which can be placed around the toilet and either bolted or, if heavy enough, allowed to stand around the toilet and held down by its own weight. To raise the toilet to the proper height for the patient to be able to use it, sometimes a raised seat attachment is adequate. Such a raised seat attachment kit can be purchased to fit any standard commode seat. If necessary to have the toilet near the patient's bed or close to the patient, a push button folding commode is available (Cleo).

BATH TUB AND SHOWER AIDS

Since frequent bathing or showering is a necessity, it is important for the bathroom to be so equipped as to encourage this activity without fear of injury and with minimum effort. To make the bathtub safe, we can place a skid-proof rubber mat on the bathtub floor. This may be purchased at any department or variety store. Or nonskid tape can be placed on the bottom of the tub. In addition, the bathtub and shower should be provided with handrails installed on the wall or on the bathtub or both. Grab bars may also be fastened to the wall with heavy duty brackets (Fig. 70 shows a typical shower, and Fig. 71, a typical bathtub). A hand brush with rubber suction cups can be attached to the sink or tub. A magic soaper for one hand use consists of

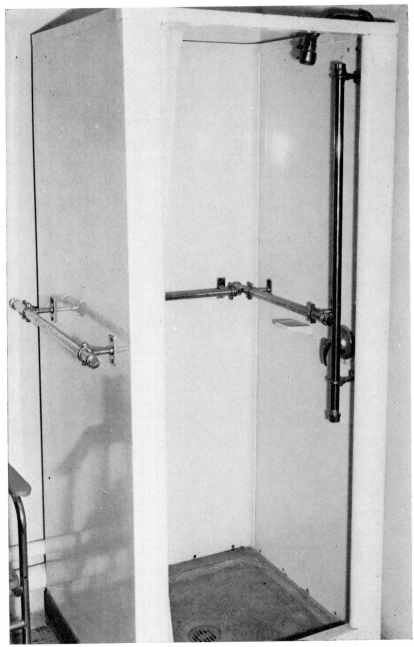

Figure 70. Typical shower; note horizontal and vertical hand rails.

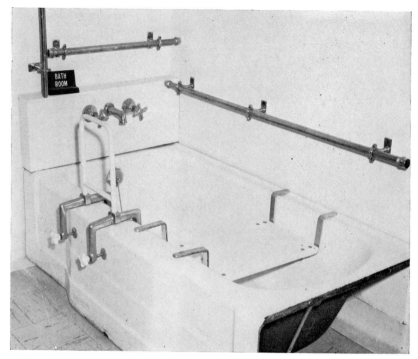

Figure 71. Typical bathtub, note bathtub seat, as well as protective rails.

a sponge in a plastic handle with provision for a bar of soap inserted in its pocket. Since it is difficult for a one-handed individual to get up from the bathtub, it is advisable to place a waterproof bath and shower bench in tub. This should have suction tips to grip tub or shower floors securely (Fig. 71).

Caution. With all the bathtub aids and conveniences it is still not advisable for the handicapped stroke patient to be in the bathtub by himself. It is strongly recommended that a member of the family or some reliable assistant be there with him.

DRESSING

Most stroke patients can be taught to dress themselves with the use of the nonparetic hand. We should however, try to help restore function in the paretic hand if only as an assist (see Chapter 12, S.A.E. routine), and in most cases we have been able to do so. But for those who have to dress with one functional hand only, there are available assistive devices to make this possible with minimal effort. Here a satisfactory teaching program by the members of the rehabilitation team is quite desirable.

Certain general rules will now be given.

1. Wherever possible use Velcro straps. They can be manipulated by one-handed individuals without much difficulty.

For those not familiar with this dressing aid, a Velcro strap consists of two nylon parts. One part is covered with hundreds of small hooks, the other part is covered with small loops. When pressed together, the hooks and loops engage and hold firmly. To disengage them one has only to pull the two parts apart. As already indicated, both of these procedures can be accomplished by a one-handed individual without much difficulty.

An interesting feature of these Velcro straps is that they can be attached to any material, limited only by the imagination. Thus they can be used on pajama tops, instead of buttons; on shoes, instead of shoe laces; and on cuffs, instead of cuff links. For the stroke patient they can be used in any area which is cosmetically acceptable to the patient.

Next to Velcro straps, probably the most useful item for the one-handed individual is the zipper. This too can be used to replace buttons such as in the crotch, on coats, blouses, and even on shoes instead of elastic shoe laces. For zippers beyond the usual reach, "zipper-pulls" are available (Cleo) that will reach all areas, front or back.

For those who wish to use regular buttons and button holes, there are now available buttoners with various sized loops. These loops are forced through the button hole, grasp the button, which is then pulled through the loop.

Dressing Routine

As a general rule, to dress, the stroke individual will hold the clothing in the nonparetic hand, first insert the paretic limb into the coat, blouse, pajama top, as the case may be, then maneuver the nonparetic limb into the garment. To undress, he will first remove the nonparetic limb from the garment.

For shoes, elastic shoe laces are now generally available that will permit the easier putting on and taking off of the shoe. A long shoe horn will obviate the need of too much bending.

Note: It is possible to teach a stroke patient to tie his shoe laces with one hand. But is it necessary with all the modern assists available? I do not think so. I do not advise it, certainly not for patients who require too much of an effort to do so.

TELEPHONING

To make it easier for the stroke patient to use the phone, several gadgets are now available. A shoulder rest can be purchased from most A. D. L. catalogues or even from ordinary mail order catalogues. The telephone is attached to this rest, and when in use, placed on the shoulder, leaving the hand free to take a message. Or the phone company will attach such a rest permanently and fit it to the individual. The telephone company will also install a speaker phone unit, which amplifies the voices at both ends by the mere push of a button on the phone.

Finally, a two-way telephone amplifier is available (Allied Radio Shack) which requires no installation. All the individual has to do is take the phone off the hook and place it on the unit. Again voices are amplified at both ends. When the conversation is finished, the phone is replaced on the hook. Other telephone assists are available, such as Luxo telephone holders or Be OK receiver holder (Be OK), for easier communication. These permit the phone to be attached to the present receiving unit, thus again leaving the hands free to write the message.

KITCHEN AIDS

The housewife with one functioning upper extremity will have to be provided with numerous assists to make life useful. These assists are now available and are constantly being added to by inventive minds.

Before discussing these aids, some general comments are in order concerning the house itself. The floor, again, should be skid-proof, by one of the methods mentioned under bathing or walking, and no loose rugs should be placed where the individual can trip. All cabinets and counters should be accessible for wheelchairs. The windows should be low and louvre type. The utensils should be electric powered, with easy-to-control on and off switches. This means an electric dish washer, electric stove, electric garbage disposal, and electric washer and dryer, and an electric iron. The ironing board should be attached to the wall for easy folding and unfolding. Again, the lamps should have either push switches or pull cords, rather than turn knobs, certainly not the small turn knobs that now come with most such lamps.

ASSISTS FOR THE HOUSEWIFE

Dressing

We already discussed some of the general dressing assists. An additional aid for the housewife is an Apron Clip (Cleo) which is made of elastic, slips in and out of the apron, and clips around the waist to hold the apron in place.

Food Preparation

A one-handed food chopper is available (Cleo) that will chop any solid or leafy food, including raw and cooked vegetables and meats. A one-handed can opener (Cleo) (Be OK) will open any can with the use of only one hand.

A jar lid opener which is attached to the wall (Be OK) can be used to open any jar by removing the screw cap; it can also be used to pry up edges and to remove bottle caps. There is also available a wall unit for removal of bottle caps which fall into a storage compartment that can be loosened and emptied at leisure.

A one-hand peeling and carving aid (Cleo) can be used to peel vegetables or fruits, or to carve a roast. It consists of a number of spears which hold the food, and a locking device which keeps it in place.

Other available aids for the one-handed housewife are described in "Homemaking Aids for the Disabled," No 710, Kenny Rehabilitation Institute, and "Do It Yourself Again," American Heart Association (Appendix C).

To test the patient's abilities as regards activities of daily living and to help train him in some of these activities, we have prepared an A. D. L. board which any member of the stroke rehabilitation team can manipulate. We have found it very useful, both for testing and training (Fig. 72).

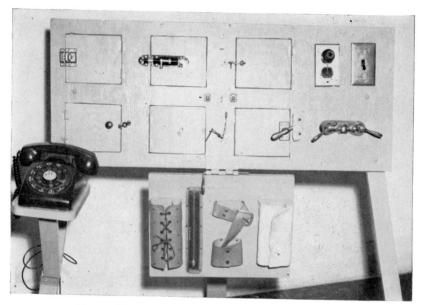

Figure 72. A.D.L. board for testing and treatment.

Having indicated the various activities of rehabilitation and daily living, let us take a typical example and thereby show some of their practical application in a given case.

CASE HISTORY, S.L.S.

Patient is a sixty-seven-year-old male admitted April 6, 1966 and discharged May 11, 1966. The history was that he was standing up by a car, and he suddenly felt weak; his left side gave way, and he slowly settled gently on the ground. Patient stated that it was obvious that he had a stroke. He did not lose consciousness. He was taken to the local hospital where it was found that his blood pressure was 140/90. At the hospital, a spinal tap showed initial pressure of 230 and closing pressure of 288 with no evidence of gross blood. He stated he had never had a similar attack, and this was the first hospitalization of his life. Family history was noncontributory. Review of systems was essentially negative. Physical examination revealed a ruddy-faced, red-nosed individual, mentally clear and cooperative. Head grossly normal with no evidence of any injury. Neck not stiff. Carotid pulses equal, no bruit. Ophthalmoscopic showed some haziness of the lens. There was slight thinning of the arterioles. Lungs clear to percussion and auscultation with slight diminution in intensity of breath sounds, left upper. Heart not enlarged. Blood pressure 125/90. The heart sounds are clear and distinct and no murmurs are heard. The peripheral vessels are sclerotic. Liver not enlarged. The extremities are normal except for paralysis of the left upper and lower extremities. The reflexes on the left are hyperactive. There is questionable Babinski. No clonus. Blood showed a hemoglobin of 13.6 gm, white count 8,950 with normal differential. Urinalysis negative except for one plus sugar. Serology negative. Fasting blood sugar 128, BUN 13, SGOT 20, SLDH 340. X-ray of the chest negative. Electrocardiogram showed a nondiagnostic tracing.

Patient was placed on a one-gram sodium diet. He was given tranquilizers and mild sedative. Under this regime, the patient got along very well. Because of the possibility of diabetes, which is not marked, the patient was placed on Orinase®, 0.5 gm twice daily and a 2000-calorie diabetic diet. He was referred to P. M. and R. service for exercise along with a foot brace for his paralyzed left foot. The patient has gotten along very well. At the present time he is able to walk with the help of a cane. However, he is still handicapped because of the weakness of the left side. He is being discharged into the care of his son and is to go to Tuskegee, Alabama where there is a Veterans Administration Hospital. Aid and attendance request was put in for the patient so he should be relieved of too much worry. Of course, patient will not be able to be employed in gainful industry.

Diagnoses

1. Arteriosclerosis, cerebral.
2. Arteriosclerosis, general.
3. Thrombosis, branch of middle cerebral, right, with left hemiplegia.

4. Diabetes mellitus, mild.

Figures 73 through 87 show some of the steps in his rehabilitation and self-care program.

Note: A list of A. D. L. references (Appendix C) and a list of sources of supply (Appendix B) will appear at end of book.

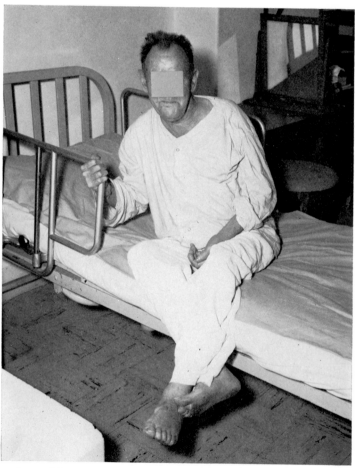

Figure 73. a. *(this page)*, b., c., and d. Patient being taught to go from bed to wheelchair.

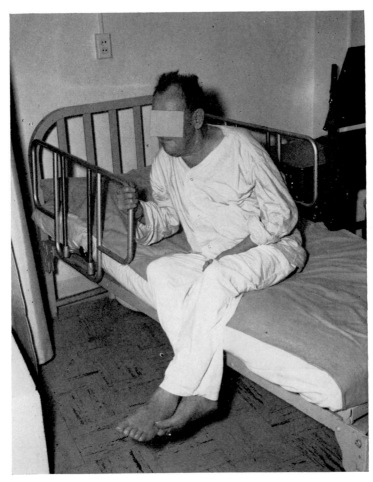

Figure 73b.

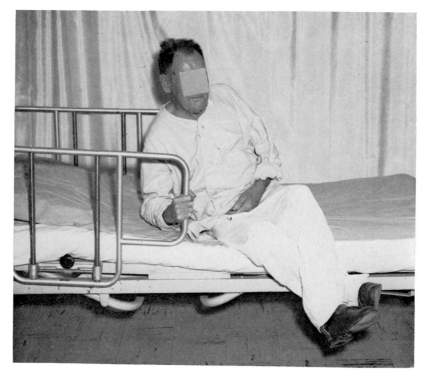

Figure 73c.

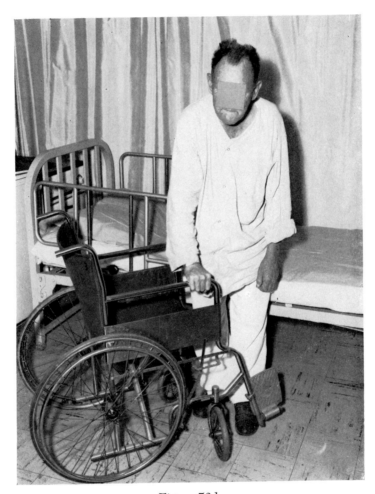

Figure 73d.

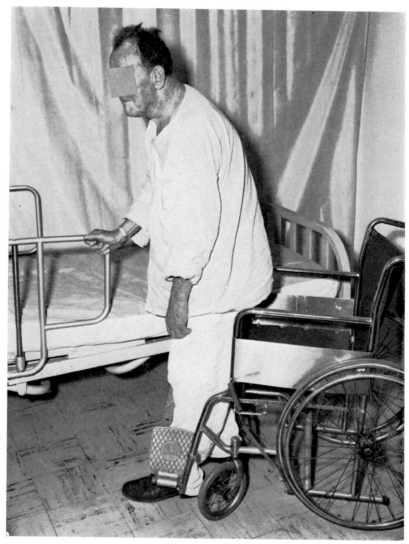

Figure 74. From wheelchair back to bed.

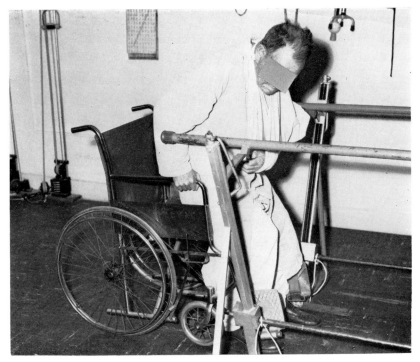

Figure 75. a. and b. From wheelchair to parallel bars.

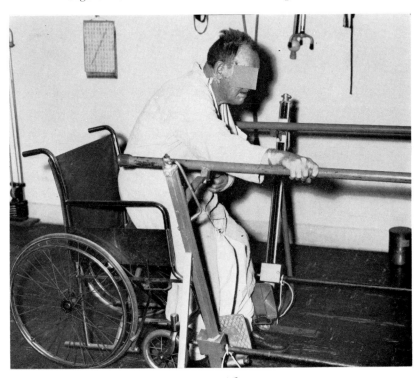

Figure 75b.

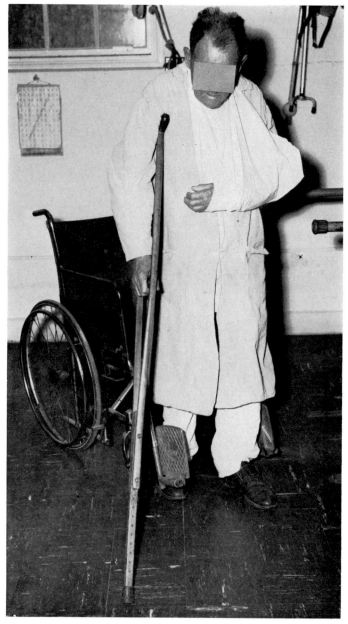

Figure 76. From wheelchair to crutch ambulation.

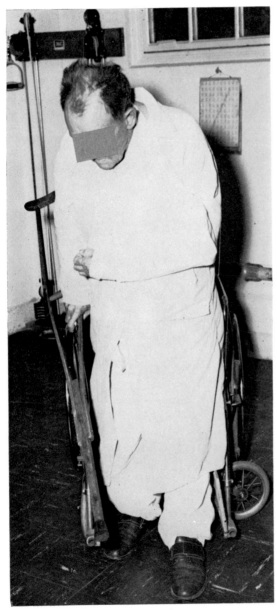

Figure 77. a, b, c, d. From wheelchair to independent cane ambulation.

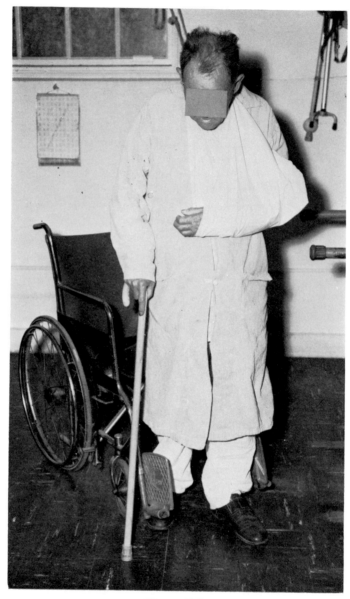

Figure 77b.

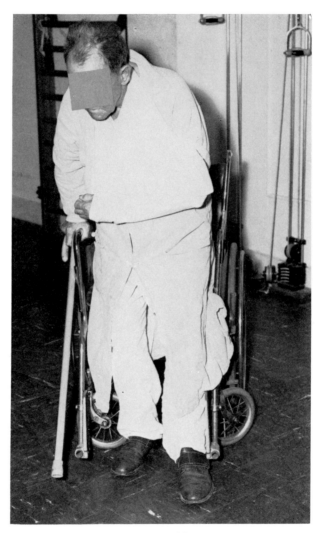

Figure 77c.

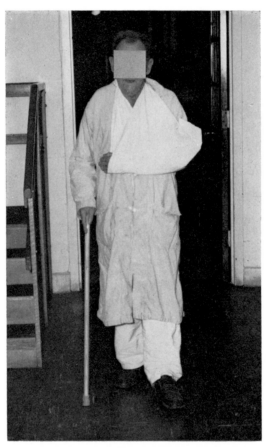

Figure 77d.

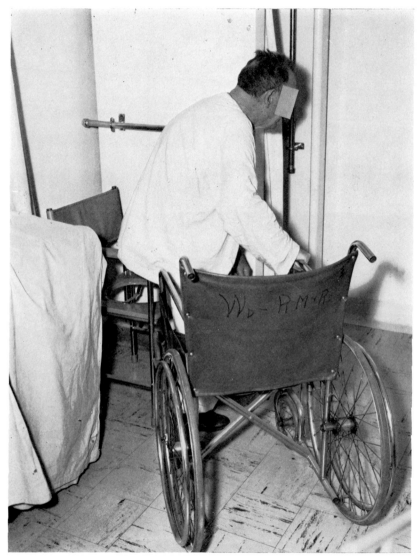

Figure 78. From wheelchair to toilet.

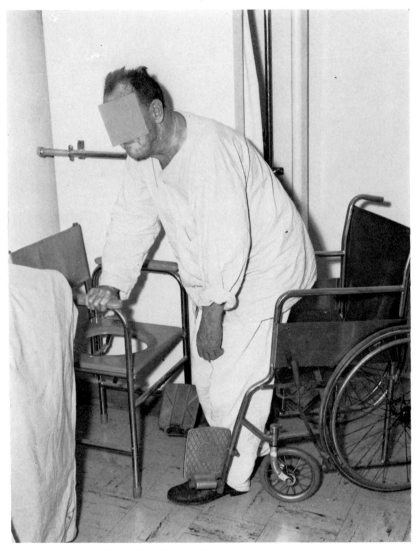

Figure 79. From toilet back to wheelchair.

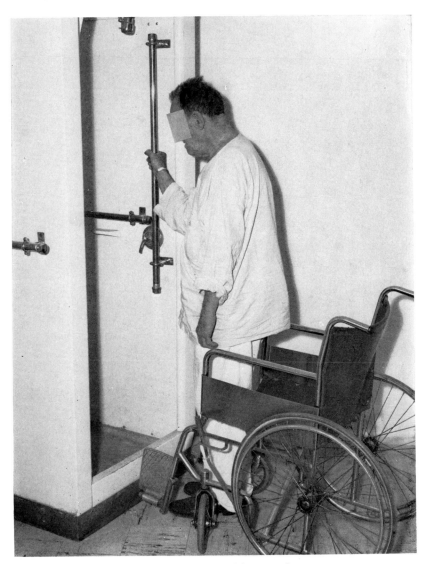

Figure 80. From wheelchair to shower.

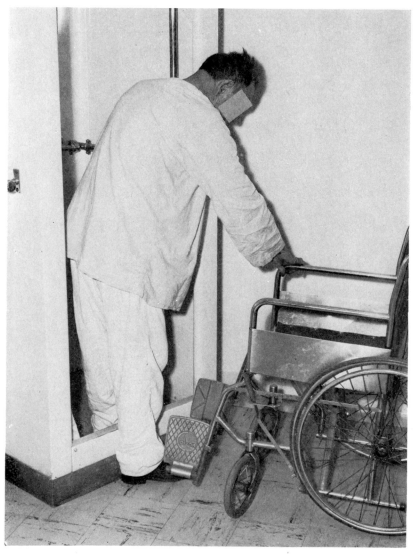

Figure 81. From shower back to wheelchair.

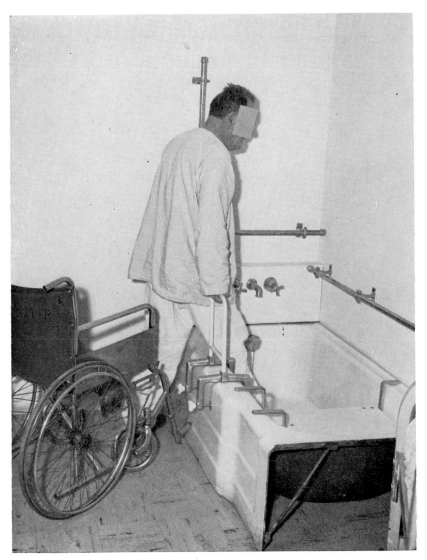

Figure 82. From wheelchair to bathtub.

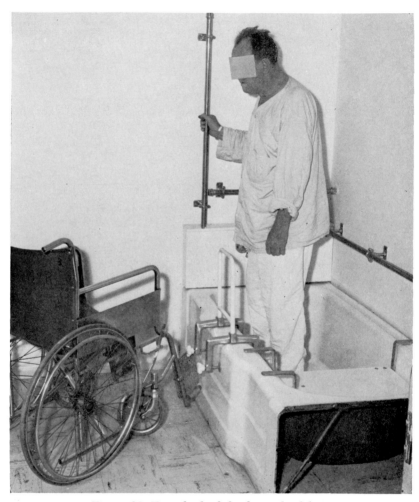

Figure 83. From bathtub back to wheelchair.

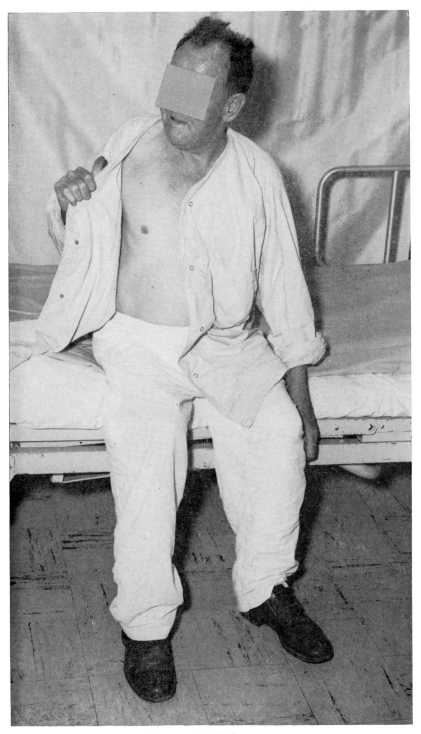

Figure 84. Undressing.

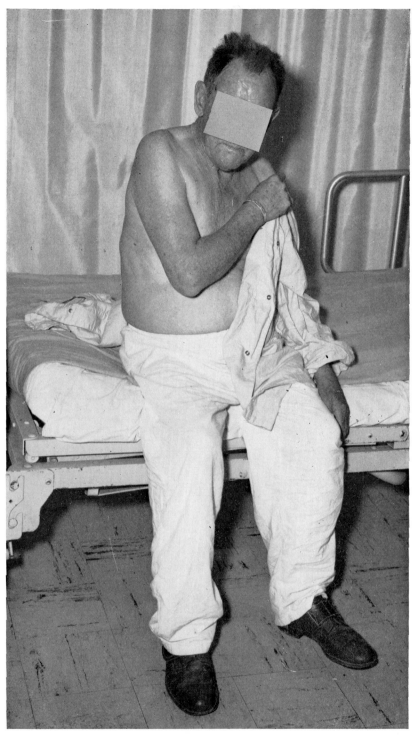

Figure 85. dressing.

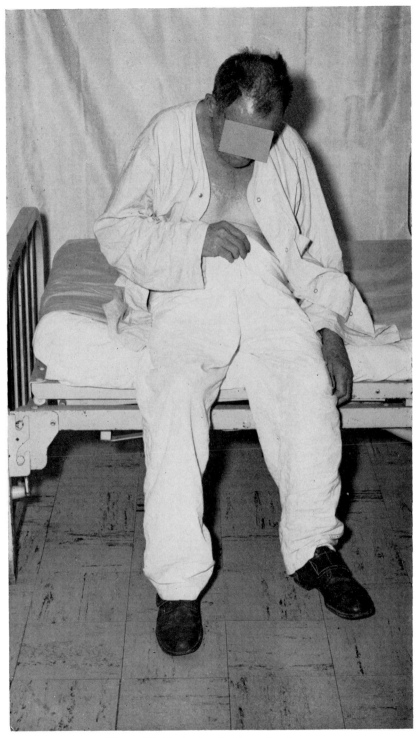

Figure 86. Buttoning bottom of pajamas.

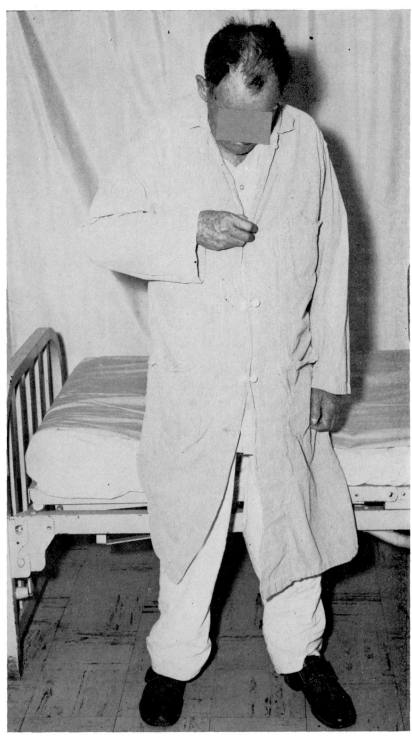

Figure 87. Buttoning robe.

PART V
THE STROKE REHABILITATION TEAM

Chapter 24

THE STROKE REHABILITATION TEAM

S EVERAL times in the last chapters, we have mentioned the stroke rehabilitation team. I cannot emphasize too strongly that if there are occasions in medicine where the doctor needs very little help from other members of the allied professions, stroke is certainly not one of them.

Here, the doctor, while medical coordinator or captain of the team, is only one member among many, including administrative coordinator, nurse, physical therapist, occupational therapist, corrective therapist, speech therapist, recreational therapist, and their rehabilitation therapy assistants, social service worker, psychologist, dietitian, volunteer, family and society, and of course, most of all the patient himself. (See Fig. 88.)

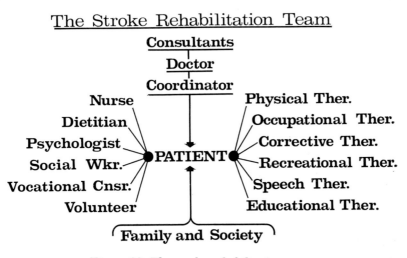

Figure 88. The stroke rehabilitation team.

FUNCTION OF THE STROKE REHABILITATION TEAM

The three salient functions of the rehabilitation team can be expressed by the acronym P.A.R.: P.—prevent, A.—assist, and R.—retrain.

Prevent

The members of the team must constantly be alert to prevent contractures, to prevent decubiti, to prevent falls, to prevent convulsions if the patient is epileptic, and to prevent injuries if a seizure occurs, and they must try to prevent atrophy from disuse. Most of these have already been discussed in previous chapters.

Assist

If the patient needs wheelchair-transfer assistance, the members of the team must help with such transfers, or if he needs supervised ambulation, they must provide such supervision and fit him with a sling for the paretic arm or a brace for a foot drop, as necessary.

Retrain

Teach the patient to walk, if possible, with or without a cane; teach him to use the nonparetic hand for writing or dressing or feeding or grooming.

Peszczynski[68] notes that encouragement, opportunity, and protection may be the basis for today's theory of rehabilitation. To these I should like to add "help," and incorporate all four into an acronym—H.O.P.E.—namely *help* where needed, but no more than needed; give the patient an *opportunity* to do things for himself, to feed himself, dress himself, comb his hair, being sure at the same time that you provide *protection* against any mishaps, and *encouragement* to cooperate with his rehabilitation program. We shall now proceed to discuss the functions of the members of this stroke rehabilitation team.

Note: The following discussion is ideal. However, as will be shown later, many of the activities mentioned are often combined and performed by a reduced team and carried out quite efficiently.

THE PATIENT

The patient is the center of the team. He is the one who is being rehabilitated. He must want to be rehabilitated or he at least must not resist it, or all the team efforts are in vain. The degree to which he will be rehabilitated depends on his age, the severity of involvement, the basic cause of his stroke, his objective, and the associated conditions.

AGE

It is generally agreed that the older the person, the more difficult the rehabilitation process. A good dividing line is the age of seventy. As a rule, patients under seventy have a better prognostic outlook than those over seventy, although, of course, there are exceptions.

Severity of Involvement

A C. V. A. associated with a severe motor or sensory involvement, or one associated with a marked dysphasia or dysmentia will not respond to our rehabilitation efforts or will respond only slightly. The aim for such patients would be maximum self-care. Usually we may have to settle for wheelchair dependency. On the other hand, a patient with a mild or moderate C.V.A., with a minor motor or sensory deficit, mild dysphasia, and minimal dysmentia, has a much better chance to get a good rehabilitation result.

Basic Cause of his Stroke

Again, it must be remembered that a stroke is an incident in a disturbed cerebrovascular system. What the disturbance is and its extent will determine the rehabilitation potential. A C.V.A. resulting from the rupture of localized berry aneurism in an otherwise fairly normal brain will yield a far more favorable result than a cerebral infarction in a brain manifesting severe cerebral arteriosclerosis. Hence, it is important to have the stroke patient examined by a neurologist or, if necessary, by a vascular or neurosurgeon in order to delineate, if possible, the cause and extent of the C.V.A.

The Objective

The objective must be realistic. It will depend upon the severity of the C.V.A. and the cause, but also on the patient's background, his prestroke social and educational and vocational history, as well as on his aim for the future. This does not mean that a patient, following a stroke, is limited by his prestroke accomplishments. A well-motivated patient with a less disabling stroke can resume where he left off and continue with this vocational plan.

One of my patients in the Veterans Administration Hospital, Cleveland, Ohio, a man of forty, developed a C. V. A. resulting in a right hemiplegia and mild dysphasia. He had indicated, before his stroke, his desire to learn Spanish. So he was referred to the educational therapy section where we had a Spanish speaking volunteer instructor. While the patient was given the usual rehabilitation activities, he was also learning Spanish. He made excellent progress. Not only did he recover from his stroke with only mild residuals, but he also obtained a job in a South American country, with our government, as a Spanish translator.

The Associated Conditions

The associated conditions will obviously affect the rehabilitation potential. Heart disease, chronic nephritis, severe arthritis, and other chronic diseases will limit the patient's ability to enter a dynamic rehabilitation program, no matter what his age. Therefore, primary attention will have to be given to them before the stroke problem is attacked.

THE PATIENT'S REACTION

The patient's reaction to his stroke is according to Metheney[69] influenced by many factors. These include the patient's age, education, intelligence, religious beliefs, cultural background, family constellation and value, and most important, the kind of person he was before the stroke. Some of the characteristics of patients that should be evaluated are the following: regression, emotional stability, overdependence, irritability, impulsiveness, depression, euphoria, apathy, hostility, self-depreciation, frustration, egocentricity, anxiety, fear, and denial of illness. Some of these manifestations have been considered in Chapter 20, "Mental Barriers."

THE DOCTOR

The doctor is captain of the stroke rehabilitation team. Preferably, he is a physiatrist, a physician specializing in physical medicine and rehabilitation. Such a physician, with his understanding of the patient's problems and of the functions of the various members of the team, will best be able medically to coordinate the functions in the best interest of the patient. Since there are not yet enough physiatrists available, then the next best thing is to find a physician of any speciality, but one who has had special training and interest in rehabilitation medicine. He could be a neurologist, internist, orthopod, or any other specialist, provided he meets these qualifications. But whatever his background, he must be the leader and supervisor of the rest of the team, or else the patient will not receive the best rehabilitation efforts possible. In addition to his professional qualifications, the doctor must be a man or woman of understanding, patience, and tact. He must certainly be alert to assess the progress of the patient and to try to determine the reasons for lack of progress; he must not just say that the patient lacks motivation.

THE COORDINATOR

In order to permit the doctor to devote his time and energy to medical and professional activities, it is advisable for the team to have the service of a lay coordinator. He can be very valuable to the team, as has been shown in many Veterans Administration Hospitals, by taking the professional load off the doctor and assuming the administrative responsibility for the entire program. He will act as liaison between the doctor and the rest of the team, be responsible for preparing statistical charts, making contacts with the community, where indicated, to provide placement for the patients who are ready for such assignments. He and the team secretary take care of the patient's records and files. He checks the progress notes for adequacy. He arranges for inservice training programs, team conferences, and rehabilitation board meetings, when the doctor feels they are needed. These men and women have proved themselves very valuable, particularly in large centers.

THE NURSE

Next to the patient and doctor, the nurse is the most important member of the stroke rehabilitation team. The nurse sees the patient, and is able to study him during most of the day and night, especially at a time when he is not under specific treatment. She notes his reaction to treatment, hears his complaints, and reports to the doctor and other team members. She should be compassionate, yet firm, be willing to do things for the patient that need to be done, and to refrain from doing things that the patient should do for himself. So often, as a PM&R consultant, have I made ward rounds and noticed that a stroke patient has an indwelling catheter far beyond the time that he needs one. On questioning the ward personnel, I have found that the nurse is too lazy or too busy to encourage the patient to void and takes the easy path of keeping the catheter in him. The stroke reha-bilitation nurse, like other members of the team, must keep up with the progress of her specialty, by reading and by attending courses in rehabilitation nursing that are now available in many rehabilitation centers. When a physical or corrective therapist is not available, the nurse, according to Schultz, must assume their functions of exercise, self-care, and ambulation.[70]

THE PHYSICAL THERAPIST

The physical therapist has been trained to test muscle func-tion, range of motion, functional evaluation, and activities of daily living. She exercises the patient as prescribed by his physician, starting with passive exercise and advancing to active assistive, active, and resistive exercise, and she supervises the S.A.E. rou-tine. In the absence of the corrective therapist, she assists the patient with transfer and self-care activities and in the absence of the occupational therapist, helps the patient with grooming. Like the nurse, she must be understanding, sympathetic, but firm. She must be very patient and often be satisfied with slow progress. She should be alert and report to the doctor any untoward re-action.

THE CORRECTIVE THERAPIST

Fortunate is the hospital that can recruit and maintain one or more corrective therapists. These men, sometimes women, are physical education graduates, many of whom have master's degrees in physical education, and who have had clinical training, usually in a Veterans Administration Hospital. They have proven themselves invaluable in the care of the patient following a stroke, particularly in the early stages, where the patient needs a strong but intelligent muscleman to help him from bed to wheelchair and back, and from wheelchair to parallel bars, and back. They too, like the nurse and physical therapist should have sympathy and understanding, and they usually do. Where they are employed, these corrective therapists will often do the testing and training for activities of daily living, including dressing, bathing, and toilet transfers, and ambulaton. Where there is no corrective therapist, I have often seen the physical therapist perform the functions of both and do an outstanding job.

THE OCCUPATIONAL THERAPIST

The occupational therapist on the stroke rehabilitation team provides purposeful activity to help the patient overcome his physical, as well as his mental disability. By careful, graded activity, she or he encourages the patient to improve function in paralyzed limbs and to utilize to the greatest potential, the limbs that are nonparetic. The occupational therapist will also help the patient by providing a shoulder sling (Fig. 89 a, b), if needed, and a wrist extension splint. (The brace-maker will usually fit the patient with a long or short leg brace, as needed, and shoulder slings can now be purchased for a nominal price.) The occupational therapist will supervise grooming activities, for the male: shaving, combing his hair, brushing his teeth; and for the female: the usual beauty parlor functions. She will also supervise feeding activities, in cooperation with the dietitian. The occupational therapist is also usually best equipped to assist the patient with self-help devices. But a good occupational therapist will do much more. He or she will encourage the patient to mingle with other patients and will be of great help in assisting with resocialization. When there is no educational therapist, the occupational thera-

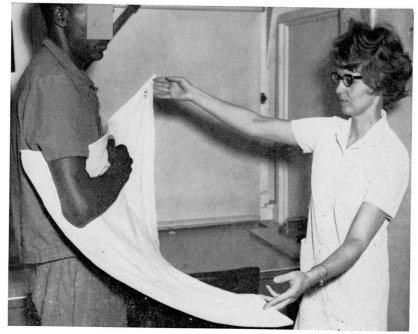

Figure 89. a. *(this page)* and b. Occupational therapist fitting shoulder sling
to patient.

pist will help the patient to learn how to use the left, nonparetic
hand, in a right hemiplegia, to write. She will encourage the
patient, by commending him for his achievements. She will sponsor arts and crafts shows by patients, in which the recreation
therapist will often participate, including hospital shows; and
arts and crafts shows by the handicapped, sponsored by the local
mayor's "employ-the-handicapped" committee, or by local busi-
nesses. The occupational therapist, as much as any other therapist, can often assume the function of an older sister as regards
taking an interest in the patient's recovery. Some of these activities are shown in Figures 90 to 100.

THE EDUCATIONAL THERAPIST

Many of the larger hospitals have educational therapists. These
men and women often have their master's degree in education.
They need indoctrination in the meaning of stroke, the symptoms

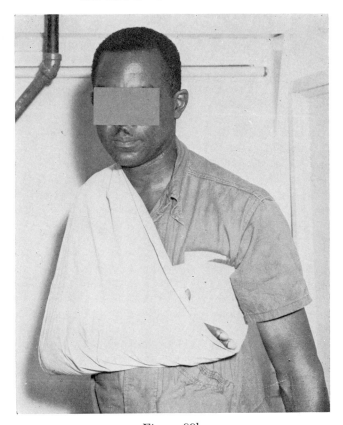

Figure 89b.

and signs. They can get this by in-service training in a hospital setting. Since they have learned the methodology of instruction, all they have to do is to apply it to a stroke-handicapped patient. I have seen them do this with good results. Often, in the absence of a speech therapist, they assume his function too. They encourage group discussion by stroke patients, including dysphasics. They sponsor current events sessions, often inviting outside speakers, thus keeping the stroke patients and other handicapped patients current with world and local events. In the younger patients, they provide the opportunity for them to take courses that will help them with future occupations. These courses are coordinated with the vocational counselor.

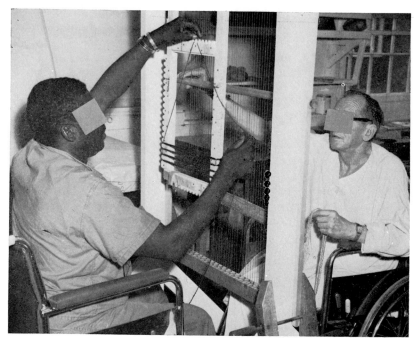

Figure 90. Patient working on hand loom in occupational therapy.

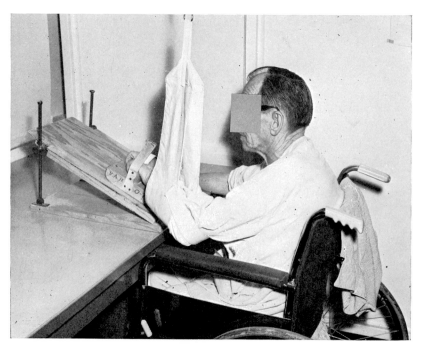

Figure 91. Patient sanding in O.T., paretic hand in sling, assisted by non-paretic hand.

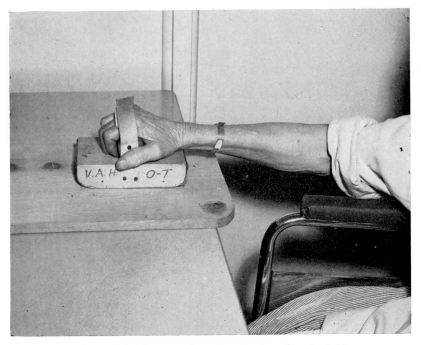

Figure 92. Close-up view of patient sanding in O.T.

THE SPEECH THERAPIST

Where a speech pathologist, a Ph.D., is available, he will assess the patient's dysphasia problem and make a speech evaluation. He will, then, supervise speech retraining, which can be given by a speech therapist, who may not have a Ph.D degree, but will have had a master's in speech, or by other members of the team. Of all the members of the team, the speech therapist probably has to have the most patience. He must not put words in the patient's mouth, but give him a chance to express himself, no matter how long it takes. It is unfortunate, but true, that many stroke patients with dysphasia make very slow progress. In fact they sometimes tend to retrogress. The speech therapist must understand, and must not react deleteriously. Furthermore, he must guide the other members of the rehabilitation team to proceed, in their patient contacts, in line with his progress. This requires

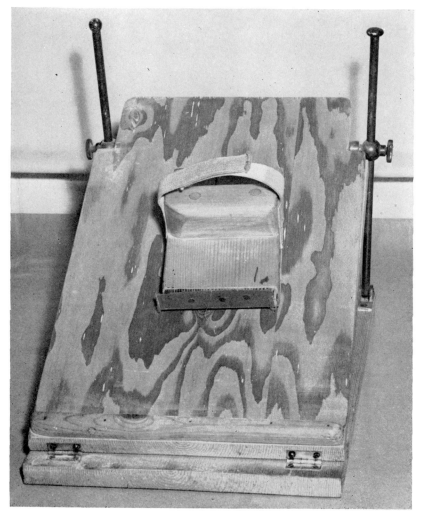

Figure 93. Sanding tool.

close team cooperation. Figure 58 shows a speech therapist trainee with dysphasia patients.

THE RECREATION LEADER

Movies, shows, parties, games, and other activities, on and off the ward, are all supervised by the recreation therapist or leader.

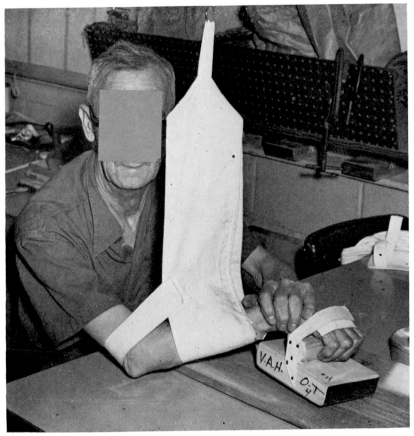

Figure 94. Patient sanding, using left (nonparetic hand) to assist right (paretic) hand which is in sling suspension.

He or she will be alert as to the patient's birthday and arrange a birthday party, to which other patients and volunteers are invited. This can be a great morale booster and a great help in resocialization. Special parties, during the Christmas season, Thanksgiving, and Halloween, with sponsorship by volunteer organizations, including veterans groups, such as: B'nai Brith, Salvation Army, American Red Cross, Music clubs, Elks, Masons, Veterans of Foreign Wars, Disabled American Veterans, and their auxiliaries, all help to bring the patients together and instill in them a feeling

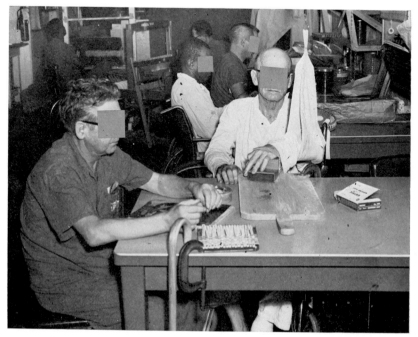

Figure 95. A group of patients undergoing treatment in O.T.

of belonging. The recreation leader is alert to community appearances by well-known groups, and gives them the opportunity to visit the hospital and provide shows for the patients. Local high school bands and church groups are always glad to help entertain patients. In summer, baseball games on adjacent diamonds are enjoyed by patients. Music therapy as a passive activity is always welcome. When the patient shows an interest, piano, organ, or guitar playing will help to restore function in the paretic hand and improve function in the nonparetic hand. Horseshoe pitching, fishing, when available, and picnics are good recreation therapy activities. Figure 101 shows arts and crafts made by patients in recreation therapy.

THE PSYCHOLOGIST

As already indicated, one of the basic problems of the stroke patient is dysmentia or disturbed mentation. While the phy-

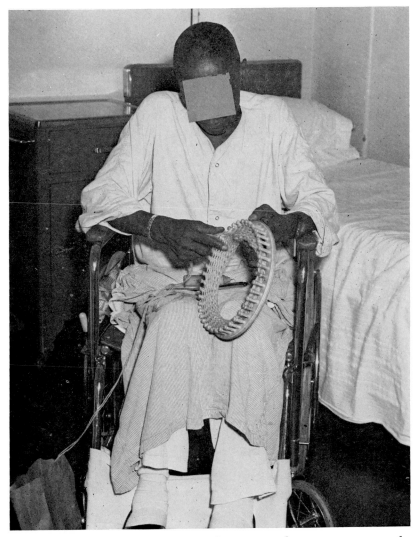

Figure 96. Patient working in O.T. with yarn to make a cap, a very popular activity.

sician and other members of the team can recognize that some difficulty exists and can usually suspect some abnormalities, it is the psychologist with his tests who can often pinpoint the exact psychological difficulty, and thus help the team to overcome it.

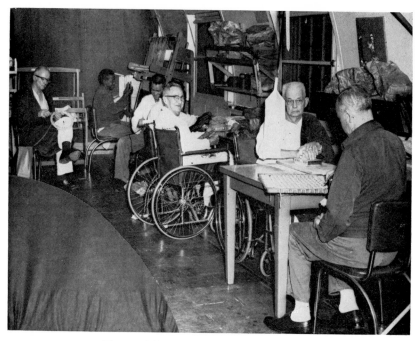

Figure 97. A group of patients in O.T.

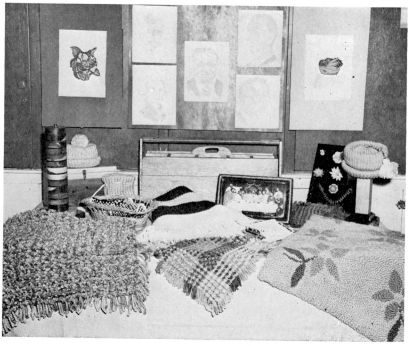

Figure 98. Some items made by patients in O.T.

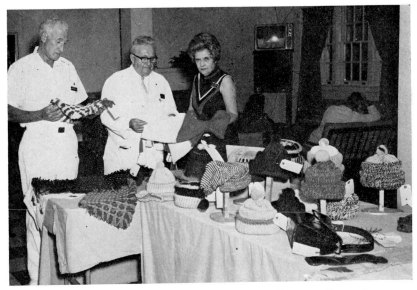

Figure 99. O.T. items displayed at annual Spring Festival.

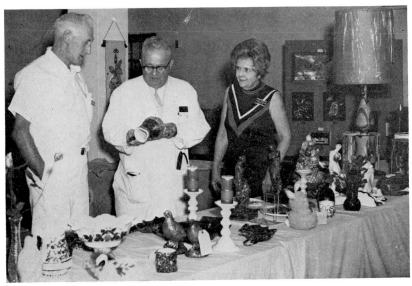

Figure 100. More items displayed at annual Spring Festival, (Note: Prizes are awarded to patients for best artifact, considering the patient's disability.)

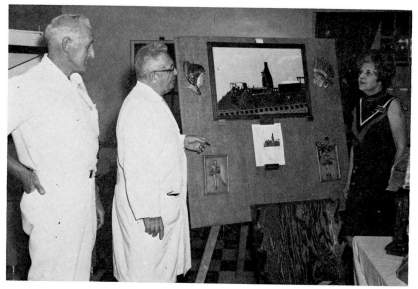

Figure 101. Arts and crafts made by patients in recreation therapy section of physical medicine rehabilitation service.

THE SOCIAL SERVICE WORKER

This team member can be of definite help by providing the rest of the team with the patient's family background and with his past social history. He also will help with discharge planning and with placement. He follows up on the patient by personal contact at home, or nursing home, to make sure that the patient is maintaining his posthospital status and not retrogressing. He arranges for placement in a nursing home, if necessary, or when the home situation is suitable, he encourages the family to take the patient home.

THE DIETITIAN

Since the patient may, and usually does, have other problems besides his stroke, it is up to the dietitian to supervise his diet under the doctor's general guidance. In addition, in cooperation with the occupational therapist, she will often help to provide special aids to the patient, so that he can enjoy and benefit by his meals. Some of these aids have been discussed in Chapter 23.

THE VOCATIONAL COUNSELOR

In younger stroke patients or in other words those who have a vocational rehabilitation potential, the vocational counselor will test the patient's aptitude, interests, and abilities, and based upon the doctor's disability assessment, will attempt to place the patient in training, in sheltered work, or in direct employment.

THE REHABILITATION THERAPY ASSISTANTS (R.T.A.'s)

Having described the functions of the various professional members of the stroke rehabilitation team, let us not forget a very important group of people who play a key role in the rehabilitation of these patients. I am considering them as a group, although we must remember that each individual in the group plays an important part in the program. By R.T.A.'s, I include P.T. assistants, O.T. assistants, C.T. assistants, R.T. assistants, S.T. assistants, and nursing assistants. As long as there is a shortage of professional personnel, and it does not look as though this shortage will be relieved for many years, R.T.A.'s will be invaluable. Nor, for that matter, does the stroke rehabilitation effort require a full cadre of professional personnel; R.T.A.'s can function very well with proper guidance and supervision. And just as there is a tendency throughout the country to train doctor's assistants to relieve the doctor's load, so I should like to see established formal training programs for these valuable people, rather than having to depend entirely on their on-the-job training. Various technical schools would be an ideal place for this purpose. Until these are established, we have to do the best we can and train these people on the job.

These men and women in physical therapy can be trained to apply Hubbard Tank, whirlpool, ultraviolet, ultrasound, infrared, passive exercise, active assistive exercise, S.A.E., active exercise, and ambulation. In occupational therapy they can be taught the usual occupational therapy modalities, including ceramics, copper tooling, leather work, printing, and handling of various looms. In speech therapy, they can assist with routine communication. In corrective theapy, they help with exercise and ambulation. In recreation therapy, they can help with R.T. activities. On the wards, they can help with all the subprofessional nurse routines, under the nurse's supervision. Needless to say, the participation of the R.T.A.'s will be limited only by their training and experience.

VOLUNTEERS

One of the most important units of the stroke rehabilitation team are the volunteers. They provide a constant exposure of the patient to the outside world. They help the patient in all other sections of his participation, including P.T., O.T., C.T., S.T., and R.T. After a brief indoctrination into their functions and in the availability of various openings, they select the area in which they are most interested, and they are assigned to that area. In the Veterans Administration Hospitals, members of the V.A.V.S., namely the Veterans Administration Volunteer Service Committee, are appointed on recommendation of local units or chapters, by their national headquarters in Washington, D.C. Together with the key members of the hospital staff, they help to formulate the programs in which the volunteers participate. The delegates to the V.A.V.S. are supposed to report back to their organizations on the various activities and on hospital patient needs. Often they will sponsor programs for patients, being responsible for bringing in talent for whom they defray the cost.

During the summer months, when high schools are closed, many senior and junior students, sponsored by the American Red Cross, volunteer for hospital duties. These junior volunteers are of inestimable value to the rehabilitation program. Like their older counterparts, they are assigned where they prefer to participate, although, being younger, they are somewhat more flexible and allow themselves to be shifted to areas where the director of volunteers feels they are most needed. For junior volunteers, these assignments are not only a chance for service, but an opportunity to observe various programs with a view, possibly, to entering some phase of the rehabilitation field. Some of the volunteers' activities are illustrated in Figures 102 to 107.

THE FAMILY AND SOCIETY

All the efforts of the entire rehabilitation team will be fruitless if the patient is not made to feel that he is wanted. Here the

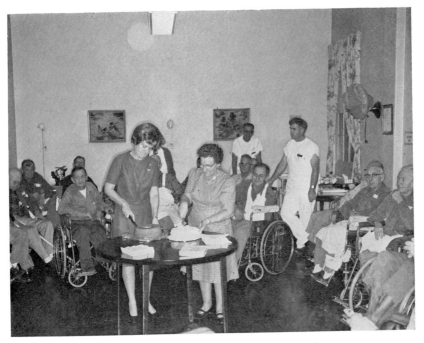

Figure 102. Birthday party sponsored by volunteers.

immediate members of his family play an important part. I have often seen a patient just give up when he comes to realize that his ever-loving wife no longer wants him at home. True, there are occasions when the wife is not able to care for a severely handicapped patient. Then the social worker will help to make other plans with the patient and his family. But I am referring to so many cases where the wife actually abandons the husband, or the husband, the wife, because the partner is no longer able to provide the companionship to which she or he has been accustomed. This is why it is so important to take the partners into our confidence early in the program and let them participate in it from the beginning. Often when the wife is convinced by actual observation that the patient, though handicapped, will not necessarily be an undue burden, she will take him home.

What is true of the family is also true, but to a lesser extent, of society. Frequent visitations by his fellow employees, his neighbors, and his minister will help the patient a great deal to maintain his interest in his rehabilitation. And nothing is a greater morale builder than for the patient to be told by his employer that his job is waiting for him.

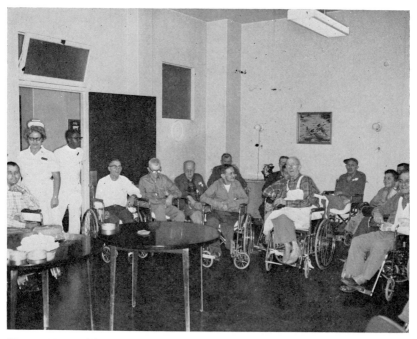

Figure 103. a. *(this page)* and b. Party sponsored by volunteers at N.H.C.U. (Nursing Home Care Unit of Columbia, South Carolina, Veterans Administration Hospital).

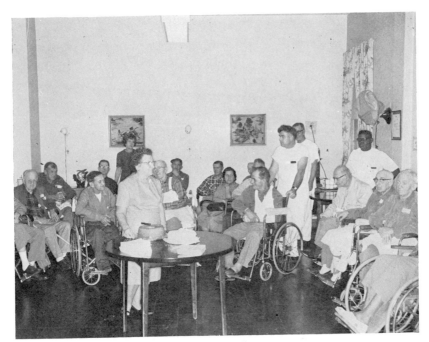

Figure 103b.

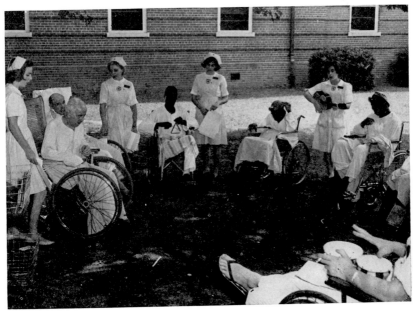

Figure 104. A group of junior volunteers entertaining patients.

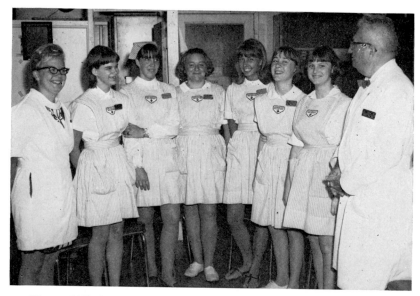

Figure 105. A group of junior volunteers photographed with author.

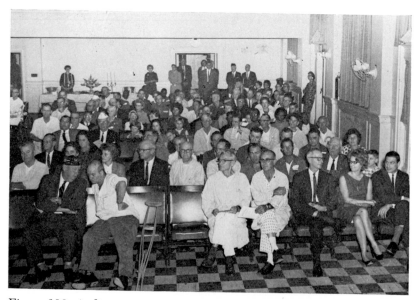

Figure 106. Audience at Annual Awards Program to honor those patients who have contributed most to their own rehabilitation.

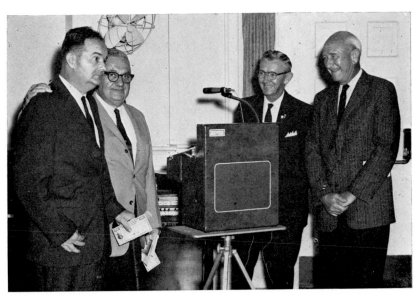

Figure 107. A stroke recovered patient holding a U.S. Government Savings Bond, at the Annual Awards Program, as one of those who had done most towards their own rehabilitation. Looking on are (right) the Director of the Veterans Administration Hospital, Columbia, South Carolina, and the Chairman of the V.A.V.S. Awards Committee, and the author, who is closest to the patient.

Chapter 25

STROKE REHABILITATION–PRESENT STATUS, AND FUTURE PROSPECTS

PRESENT STATUS

I N the preceding chapters, the reader has been given an idea of what is being done with respect to the rehabilitation of a patient following a stroke. We have indicated the possible etiologic factors, the pathophysiology, the various methods of evaluation, the stroke 4-dys syndrome and its management, the barriers, and special problems. We have reviewed the requirements for a stroke patient to lead a useful existence, including an enumeration of some commonly used self-help devices. And we have discussed the composition of an ideal stroke rehabilitation team, and the functions of each of its members.

It is unfortunate that while we now have sufficient knowledge to assist the stroke patient to attain his maximum usefulness, we do not always apply this knowledge. This happens to be true not only in most nursing homes but also in many hospitals.

Too many hospitals feel that their function is ended when they have admitted a stroke patient, made a definitive diagnosis, administered appropriate treatment, and saved the patient's life. Too many nursing homes feel that, as one administrator put it, "This is the end of the road." For most nursing home patients, this is just what it is.

Therefore, before we discuss future prospects, let us attempt to utilize our present knowledge (a) to restore maximum function to the stroke patient, and (b) to teach him to lead a useful existence with what he has left.

I hope that the previous chapters have given the reader an idea of what can be done, with a good rehabilitation team. Nor do I mean to imply that in each case, the services of all members

256

of the team are necessary or even desirable. In each case, the doctor must decide what the patient can hope to accomplish and prescribe those activities which will help him to achieve this goal. Very often, the doctor, the nurse, possibly with the help of a physical therapist, can meet the rehabilitation needs of the stroke patient. I am assuming that a sufficient number of R.T.A.'s (rehabilitation therapy assistants), will be available to supplement this abbreviated team. However, for the severely disabled stroke patient, the entire team, or a great part of it is not only desirable but necessary.

The Veterans Administration, in which I served for many years as Chief of Physical Medicine Rehabilitation in various hospitals, has shown what can be done with a good rehabilitation program. In my last hospital (Veterans Administration Hospital, Columbia, South Carolina,) an analysis of 500 stroke patients over a ten-year period[52] revealed that 132 patients became ambulatory with or without a foot-drop brace, 145 became ambulatory with a crutch or cane, 67 had to be satisfied with wheelchair independence, and 110 remained bedridden or wheelchair dependent. These results, it should be emphasized, were obtained with patients in the older group. (46 died)

It is true that only eight of one hundred consecutive patients showed a complete recovery from their dysphasia, fifty could communicate but with some difficulty, and 42 could not communicate at all. These results it should be remembered were obtained by a full-time speech therapist.

Comparing results of management of stroke patients in the years 1948 to 1956 (736 patients), with the years 1959 to 1963, (777 patients), Adams[71] reported that the prospects for stroke patients have improved. He concluded, however, that survival depended entirely on the underlying arterial disease, and that there is no way to change the course of this disease at this time.

Boyle and Scalzitti[72] studied 478 patients referred to the Department of PM&R of the Milwaukee County Hospital, of a total of 669 patients with cerebrovascular accidents admitted to this hospital. Their results were as follows: seventy (35.6%) died during their first admission, and sixty-three (13.2%) were able to perform the activities of daily living without limitation. Of the patients who expired, many had more physical and occupational therapy sessions than those who survived and were rehabilitated. From this observation, they concluded that there is no apparent relationship between the number of physical therapy and occupational therapy treatments and the ability of patients to be successfully rehabilitated. It seems to me that it would be more accurate to say that there is no relationship between the survival of stroke patients and their demise, with the number of physical therapy and occupational therapy treatments. I do not believe that we can claim that physical therapy or occupational therapy or the two together will prevent an acute stroke patient from dying. What I do believe is that if the patient survives his acute stroke, then a good rehabilitation program will result in a better functioning patient than a poor program or no program.

FUTURE PROSPECTS

According to Public Health Service Statistics,[73] 21 percent of stroke patients die after an initial attack of cerebral thrombosis, and of the 79 percent who survive the first stroke, fifty percent die in four years. Therefore, the first step in stroke management is to try to reduce the incidence of cerebrovascular accidents; the second step is to strive for a reduction in mortality from the first stroke, and the third step is to work towards a reduction of stroke recurrences. If these latter two steps are achieved, we may then finally hope to return more patients to maximum usefulness.

We know now, that certain predisposing factors tend to produce a cerebral thrombosis, namely, atherosclerosis, hyperlipidemia, uncontrolled hypertension, severe diabetes, and excess obesity. We also believe that cigarette smoking may play some part in stroke production. As we learn more how to prevent and control these factors, we may reasonably expect that the incidence of stroke will be reduced. Since this manual deals primarily with rehabilitation, we, that is the rehabilitation team, should try to utilize our present knowledge and should be alert to prevent repeated strokes. It is anticipated that, as times goes on, the prospects for this preventive program will be improved.

Specifially, newer and better techniques will be developed to study the anatomy and physiology of the extracerebral, and intracerebral arteries, and capillaries, as well as arteriovenous malformations which so often are the cause of intracerebral bleeding. Better methods will no doubt be found to manage these abnormalities.

As far as we know, only the larger cerebral arteries have been shown to have smooth muscle fibers supplied by nerve fibers, and only these larger arteries can go into vasospasm. I should not be surprised if, in time, smaller arterioles will be shown to have innervated smooth muscle, and that spasm of these smaller arterioles may also be responsible for stroke production. In time, also, methods will be found to reduce this spasm, and thus to prevent strokes.

It is anticipated that, in the future, improved blood flow recording instruments and techniques will enable us better to study cerebral blood flow in animals as well as man, and that better drugs and physical modalities will be developed to improve such blood flow, where indicated. In this respect, Liberson[74] comments that rheoencephalography, by recording intracerebral impedence, will allow us to investigate cerebrovascular changes and will thus contribute to the study of cerebrovascular lesions.

Echoencephalography, i.e. brain scanning by means of ultrasonation, has been coming into increasing use to localize those brain structures that normally occupy the midline. Specifically, it will be used with greater frequency to help delineate cerebral hemorrhage and subdural hematoma versus cerebral thrombosis and embolism.

Better devices and techniques will be developed for measuring arterial parameters in the brain by electroencephalography, echoencephalography, and arteriography with contrast and radioactive media.

In the management of the acute stroke patient, further advances may be anticipated, including the devolopment of newer anticoagulants to dissolve blood clots and fibrin. Improved techniques will be used to prevent and treat acute strokes of intracerebral, as well as extracerebral origin, and to prevent their recurrences.

What about the future prospects for surgery in the treatment of spasticity and contractures? In a recent article, Treanor,[75] reported on seven hundred surgical patients operated on for orthopedic complications following a stroke. He recommends that surgical methods be used more often to modify individual parameters of the hemiplegic posture. For stroke patients with such complications, it is likely that more of them, particularly the younger patients, able to undergo surgery, will be referred to orthopods for these procedures.

As regards rehabilitation, we may expect to see a whole new set of electronic devices to assist patients with ambulation and self-care. Newer methods will be produced to measure and treat spasticity and incoordination, and to assess smaller gradations of strength and range of motion, and better equipment and techniques will be developed to improve them.

As knowledge of the management of stroke patients increases and its dissemination is widened we can hope and expect that professional and public apathy towards rehabilitation will be abated and that the community will thus be motivated to insist that every effort be made not only to save the patient's life, but also to make that life more meaningful.

More and better community pilot stroke programs, such as those now sponsored by the various state regional medical units, as well as by many rehabilitation centers, will help to foster such improved techniques and make them available to all.

REFERENCES

1. United States Department of Health, Education, and Welfare: *Monthly Vital Statistics*. vol. 14, no. 13, July 15, 1966.

2. United States President's Commission on Heart Disease, Cancer, and Stroke: *Report to the President*. Washington, D.C., United States Government Printing Office, 1964, and 1965, vol. II.

3. United States National Office of Vital Statistics: *Vital Statistics in the United States*, 1958, section 8.

4. Goldberg, I. D., and Curland, L. T.: Mortality in 33 countries from diseases of the nervous system. *World Neurol*, 3:444-465, 1962.

5. Katsuki, S., Hirota, Y., Akazome, T., Takeya, S., and Takano, S.: Epidemiological studies of cerebrovascular diseases in Hasayman, Kyushu Island, Japan, part I. *Jap Heart J*, 5:12-36, 1964.

6. Kannel, W. B., Dawber, T. R., and McNamara: Vascular diseases of the brain-epidemiologic aspects: The Framingham study. *Amer J Public Health*, 55:9, 1965.

7. Metropolitan Life Insurance Company: *Statistical Bulletin*. 1964, vol. 45.

8. United States Department of Health, Education and Welfare, National Health Center for Health Statistics: Series 12, No. 8, 1964.

9. Heart and Circulation, Second National Conference on Cardio-Vascular Diseases. vol. 1, p. 18, research p. 423.

10. Robinson, R. W. *et al.*: Life table analysis for survival after cerebral thrombosis, ten years experience: JAMA, *169 L*: 1149-1152, 1959.

11. Fisher, M.: Occlusion of carotid arteries. *Arch Neurol Psychiat*, 72: 187-204, 1954.

12. Page, I. H.: *A Study of Concepts in Proceedings of National Stroke Congress*. Springfield, Thomas, pp. 37-44.

13. Lyons, C.: *Proceedings of National Stroke Congress*. Springfield, C Thomas, 1966, p. 36.

14. Hazell, K.: *Social and Medical Problems of the Elderly*, 2nd ed. Springfield, Thomas, 1966, pp. 122-139.

15. *A Classification and Outline of Cerebrovascular Diseases:* A Report of the Ad Hoc Committee established by the Advisory Council for the Institute of Neurological Diseases and Blindness, Public Health Service. Neurology, vol. 8, no. 5, 1958.

16. Toole, J. F.: *Diagnosis and Management of Stroke*. American Heart Association, 1965.

17. Vasuka, F. A.: *Essentials of the Neurological Examination*. Philadelphia, Smith, Kline, and French Laboratories, 1962.

18. Dinken, H.: Evaluation of disability and treatment in hemiplegia. *Arch Phys Med, 28*:263, 1947.

19. Deaver, G. G., and Brown, M. E.: *Physical Demands of Daily Life: An Objective Scale of Rating the Orthopedically Exceptional.* New York, The Institute of Crippled and Disabled, 1945.

20. Thomas, S. W., Izutsu, S., and Spangler, D. P.: *A Thomasat Manual, A Test for Evaluating Motor Skills of Upper Extremities.* Highland View Hospital, Cleveland, Ohio, 1957.

21. Thomas, S. W., Spangler, D. P., Izutsu, S., and Peszczynski, M.: An analysis of psychomotor responses of adult hemiplegic patients. *Arch Phys Med, 42*:85, 1961.

22. The Institute of Crippled and Disabled: *Testing, Orientation, and Work Evaluation in Rehabilitation.* New York, 1957.

23. Rusk, H. A.: *Hemiplegia and Rehabilitation.* Institute of Physical Medicine and Rehabilitation, 1952.

24. Shoening, A., Aderegg, L., Bergstrom, D., Fonda, M., Steinke, N., and Ulrich, P.: Numerical scoring of self-care status of patients. *Arch Phys Med, 46*:10, 689-697, 1965.

25. Fulton, J. F., and Sheehan, D.: The uncrossed lateral pyramidal tract in higher primates. *J Anat 69*:181-187, 1935.

26. Marks, M.: Gait Analysis of the hemiplegic patient, force plate and strobocobic studies, quarterly review. *Pediatrics. 7*:5, 1959.

27. Weldon, G. B.: Metabolic effects of immobilization. *Proceedings of First and Second Medical Conference on M.D.A.,* 1951-1959.

28. Dock, W.: Undesirable effects of bed rest. *Surg Clin N Amer 25*: 437-441, 1945.

29. Keys, A.: *Physiology of Exercise in Relation to Physical Medicine.* 1945, Vol. 26, pp. 633-638.

30. Perry, J.: Orthopedic management of the lower extremity in hemiplegic patients. *J Amer Phys Ther Ass, 46*:4, 345, 1966.

31. Samberg, H. H.: Two-buckle T-strap, a modification of the conventional T-strap. *Arch Phys Med, 50*:5, 290-291, 1969.

32. Peszczynski, M.: The intermittent double step gait. *Arch Phys Med, 39*:494, 1958.

33. Bard, G., and Ralson, H. J.: Measurement of energy expenditure during ambulation with special reference to evaluation of assistive devices. *Arch Phys Med, 40*:415, 1959.

34: Kabat, H.: Proprioceptive facilitation in therapeutic exercise. In Licht, Sidney (Ed.): *Therapeutic Exercise.* 1950, Library of Physical Medicine, Elizabeth Licht.

35. Fay, T.: The use of pathological and unlocking reflexes in the rehabilitation of spastics. *Amer J Phys Med, 33*:347, 1954.

36. Bobath, K., and Bobath, B.: Control of Motor Function in the Treatment of Cerebral Palsy. *Physiotherapy, 43*:295-303, 1957.

37. Rood, M. S.: Neurophysiological mechanisms utilized in the treatment of muscular dysfunction. *Amer J Occup Ther, 10*:220-224, 1956.

38. Psaki, R. C., and Treanor, W. J.: Afferent influence in the management of spastic paresis. *Arch Phys Med, 37*:4, 214-218, 1956.

39. Zankel, H. T.: Stimulation assistive exercise in hemiplegia (S. A. E.). *Geriatrics, 15*:616-622, 1960.

40. Holmes, G.: Clinical symptoms of cerebellar disease and their interpretation. Lancet, *1*:1177-1182, 1231-1237; *2*:59-65, 111-115, 1922.

41. Peele, T.: *The Neuroanatomical Basis of Clinical Neurology.* New York, McGraw Hill, 1954, pp. 269-273.

42. Herman, R.: The physiologic basis of tone, spasticity and rigidity. *Arch Phys Med, 43*:108-114, 1962.

43. Khalili, A. A.: Pathophysiology, clinical picture, and management of spasticity. In *Neurologic Considerations.* F. A. Davis Co., 1967, chap. 5, pp. 132-136.

44. Takamari, M.: H reflex study in upper motor neuron disease. *Neurology, 17*:32, 1967.

45. Zankel, H. T.: Effect of compression, cold, ultrasound on conduction velocity of the ulnar nerve. *Arch Phys Med, 47*:787, 1966.

46. Tigney, D. R. L., and Sheldon, K. W.: Simultaneous use of heat and cold in the treatment of muscle spasm. *Arch Phys Med, 43*:235, 1962.

47. Newton, M. J., and Lehmkuhl, D.: Muscle spindle response to body heating and localized muscle cooling: Implication for relief of spasticity. *J Amer Phys Ther Ass, 45*:91, 1965.

48. Negrin, J., Jr.: Local hypothermia in the spinal cord for relief of spasticity and rigidity, preliminary observations, *Arch Phys Med, 47*:169, 1966.

49. Lee, W. J., *et al.*: Continuous tetanizing currents for relief of spasticity and rigidity, preliminary observations. *Arch Phys Med, 31*:766, 1950.

50. Zankel, H. T.: Pallesthesia studies in stroke patients. *Southern Med J, 62*:1, 8-11, 1969.

51. Wepman, J. M.: *Recovery From Aphasia.* New York, Ronald Press Company, 1951, p. 30.

52. Zankel, H. T., Cobb, J. B., and Huskey, F. E.: The rehabilitation of 500 stroke patients. *J Amer Geriat Soc, 14*:11, 1966.

53. Wepman, J. M., and Jones, L. V.: *Studies in Aphasia,* Chicago, Education in Industry Service, 1961.

54. Schuel, H., Jenkins, J. J., and Jimenis, P. E.: Aphasia in Adults, New York, Paul E. Hoeber, Inc., 1964.

55. Porch, B.: Porch Index of Communicative Ability. Palo Alto, California, Consulting Psychologists Press, 1967.

56. Eisenson, Jon: *Examining For Aphasia.* New York, The Psychological Corporation, 1954.

57. Sands, E., Sarno, M. T., and Shakweiler, D.: Long term assessment of language function due to stroke. *Arch Phys Med, 50*:202-206, 1969.

58. Liberson, W .T.: Study of evoked potentials in aphasia. *Amer J Phys Med, 45*:3, 135-142, 1966.

59. Kottke, F. J.: The specialist role in continuing care of the stroke patient. In *Proceedings of the National Stroke Congress*. Springfield, Thomas, 1964, pp. 128-130.

60. Kosiak, M.: An effective method of preventing decubital ulcers. *Arch Phys Med, 47*:11, 725, 1966.

61. Weinstein, J. D., and Davidson, B. A.: A fluid-support mattress and seat for the prevention and treatment of decubitus ulcers. *Lancet,* pp. 625-626, 1965.

62. Allison, R. S.: *The Senile Brain.* London, William Wilkings, 1962.

63. Adams, G. F., and Hurwitz, L. J.: Mental barriers to recovery from stroke. *Lancet, 2*:533ff, 1963.

64. Bruell, J. H., and Peszczynski, M.: Perception of verticality in hemiplegic patients in relation to rehabilitation. *Clin Orthop,* no. 12, 1958.

65. Birch, H. G., Proctor, F., Bortner, M., and Lowenthal, M.: Perception in hemiplegia, judgement in the median plane. *Arch Phys Med, 41*:19, 1960.

66. Birch, H. G., Belmont, I., Reilley, T., and Belmont, L: Visual verticality in hemiplegia. *Arch Neurol 5*: 444-453, 1961.

67. Belmont, I.: Effect of cerebral damage on motivation in rehabilitation. *Arch Phys Med, 50*:507-511, 1969.

68. Peszczynski, M.: Rehabilitation of the adult hemiplegic. In *Locomotor System, Fourth Annual Volume of Physiology and Experimental Sciences.* Calcutta, India, 1963.

69. Metheney, R. V.: The nursing clinics of north America, *Chronic Rehab,* pp. 443-449, 1966.

70. Schultz, L. C. M.: The nursing care of patients with stroke. *Alabama J Med Sci, 5*:1, 28-32, 1968.

71. Adams, G. F.: Prospects for patients with strokes, with special reference to hypertensive hemiplegics. *Brit Med J 2*:253-259, 1965.

72. Boyle, R., and Scalzitti, P. D.: A study of 480 cases of cerebrovascular accident. *Arch Phys Med, 44*:1, 19-29, 1963.

73. Department of Health, Education, and Welfare, Public Health Service: *Understanding the Brain and Nervous System,* Publication no. 962, pp. 66-76.

74. Liberson, W. T.: Electroencephalography. *Amer J Psychiat, 119*:609, 1963.

75. Treanor, W. J.: The role of physical medicine treatment in stroke rehabilitation. *Clin Ortho, 63*:14-18, 1969.

APPENDIX A

INTRODUCTION

In order to spread the gospel of stroke rehabilitation possibilities, I have written what I call a "phystheatric demonstration" on stroke rehabilitation and have produced it on several occasions. These have been sponsored by interested lay organizations, usually in connection with the President's Employ-the-Handicapped Week (the first week in October). I have produced these in Cleveland, Ohio; Durham, North Carolina; and Columbia, South Carolina. I have found the Veterans Administration Voluntary Service Advisory Committee of the Veterans Administration Hospitals perfectly willing to sponsor these programs, and to donate awards to those patients who have done most for their own rehabilitation.

While in Durham, North Carolina, as Chief of Physical Medicine and Rehabilitation of the Veterans Administration Hospital, I presented such a demonstration at WUNC-TV, Chapel Hill, North Carolina. This was a true story of a patient who had obtained a good rehabilitation result following a stroke. I used the PM&R staff as participants, and the Chief of Corrective Therapy was the "patient" during the demonstration, that is, until the very end of the program when I brought out the real patient and presented him to the viewing audience.

A copy of this "phystheatric demonstration" follows. I called it *From Bed to Job*. It was presented at WUNC-TV, October 9, 1959, 8:00 to 8:30 P.M.

With slight modifications, it can be presented by a stroke rehabilitation team on television or before a live audience.

FROM BED TO JOB

HARRY T. ZANKEL

Announcer. This is National Employ-the-Handicapped Week. In this connection and to encourage employers to hire handicapped, we are pleased to present the true story of a patient suffering from a stroke and how, through a program of rehabilitation, he was restored to society, literally "from bed to job." The title of this dramatization is *From Bed to Job*. It was written by Dr. Harry T. Zankel, Chief, Physical Medicine and Rehabilitation Service of the Veterans Administration Hospital in Durham, and will be presented by Dr. Zankel and other members of the Physical Medicine and Rehabilitation Service of that hospital. So here is Dr. Zankel to tell us about this patient with hemiplegia. Dr. Zankel.

265

Dr. Zankel. Thank you, Mr. "A." "Hemiplegia" *(pointing to blackboard on which is spelled the word "hemiplegia").* "Hemi"—half, "plegia"—paralysis. A paralysis of one half of the body, right half or left half, face, arm and leg. Sometimes associated with loss of ability to communicate *(points to blackboard),* "aphasia" or "dysphasia," literally "a"—without, "phasia"—speech; or "dys—difficulty with, "phasia"—speech. The causes are many blows on the head, wounds, but most commonly *(points to blackboard)* "cerebrovascular accident." "Cerebro—brain, "vascular"—blood vessel, what is commonly known as a stroke. Such was the case of Jack Lynn. Jack is forty years old, single, lives with his sister; Second World War veteran; owns a small country store. Last December 17, Jack was about to get up to go to work as usual, but he couldn't move his leg. He tried to call his sister; his mouth opened, but no sound. In desperation he tried to get out of bed and fell to the floor. Doctor—ambulance, and Jack was taken to the hospital—the usual examination, emergency treatment, x-rays, EKG, laboratory tests. Diagnosis—thrombosis of left middle cerebral artery, right hemiplegia, and aphasis—a stroke. Now comes the long up-hill struggle for rehabilitation.

SCENE 2

Patient in bed—Dr. X listening to his heart.

Dr. Zankel. Here he is in bed; posture is good. There is a pillow between right arm and side to keep the muscles from contracting. Notice the foot-drop board to keep the right foot from falling forward, and the sand bag on the side to keep the foot from dropping to one side. Dr. X, Assistant Chief, Physical Medicine and Rehabilitation, is just finishing his examination.

(Dr. X puts stethoscope in pocket.)

Dr. X. Now Mr. Lynn, let's see what you can do. *(He raises his left leg.)* Hold it *(patient does so); now let it go. (He does.)* Now I'll raise the right arm. *(He does so.)* Hold it. *(Patient drops it.)* Now your right leg. *(Doctor raises it.)* Hold it. *(Patient can't; it falls like a dead weight).* Now Mr. Lynn, let's see you raise your left arm. *(Patient does so.)* Down *(obeys).* Now lift *left* leg *(obeys).* Down *(obeys).* Now your *right* arm, please. *(Patient raises his* left *arm.)* I said your *right* arm. *(Doctor holds left arm down; patient does not move either arm.)* Now *(doctor holds left leg down)* raise your right leg. *(patient attempts to raise left leg.)* Now, Mr. Lynn, I am going to send a physical therapist here to give you some exercise. Later we shall call you to the clinic, O.K.?

(Patient nods.)

SCENE 3

Back to Dr. Zankel.

Dr. Zankel. Physical therapy is started early on these patients—range of motion exercises, massage. Suppose we show you. Here is Miss Y, one of our physical therapists.

SCENE 4

Shifts back to previous scene, Miss Y at bedside.

Miss Y. Now, Mr. Lynn, all you have to do is relax. I'll do the rest. I shall put each of your joints through its range of motion. First your shoulder *(she does so)*, now your elbow *(she does so)*, now your wrist *(she does so)*, and your fingers *(she does so)*, now your hip *(she does)*, your knee *(she does)*, your ankle *(she does)*, your foot and toes *(she does)*. Now I shall massage your leg *(she does)*, from foot to knee to help the circulation.

SCENE 5

Shifts back to Dr. Zankel.

Dr. Zankel. And from now until discharge P.T. will have something to do with this patient. Range of motion exercise, massage, neuromuscular reeducation. But let's go on with our story. A month has passed. Miss Y has seen the patient daily; the nurses have given the usual excellent nursing care; the doctors have watched him all this time; people have been doing things for the patient, but now the time has come for Mr. Lynn to do things for himself. So now we find him in the A.D.L.—activities of daily living section.

SCENE 6

Shifts to A.D.L. section, A.D.L. board to one side.

The patient is in a wheelchair, right foot in drop foot brace.

Dr. Zankel. Remember how flaccid he was last time we saw him? Look at him now. Right arm is becoming spastic. Notice the foot drop brace. As to speech, well, we'll soon find out as Mrs. Z, Chief, Occupational Therapy, teaches him the fundamentals of A.D.L., activities of daily living. *(Mrs. Z walks in).*

Mrs. Z. My name is Mrs. Z. I'm the Chief, Occupational Therapy. What's your name?

Patient. Ah, ah.

Mrs. Z. Jack Lynn?

Patient. Ah, ah.

Mrs. Z. How old are you?

Patient. Ah, ah.

Mrs. Z. You're doing fine.

Patient. (Points to A.D.L. board.) Eh?

Mrs. Z. This is called an A.D.L. board—activities of daily living. Let's see what you can do with it. But first I think we ought to do something about your hair. *(Hair is disheveled.)* Have you got a comb? *(He struggles for a comb and pulls it out of pajama pocket.)*

Patient. (Triumphantly) Ug. *(He wants to put it back in his pocket, Mrs. Z stops him.)* OK, why don't you use it? *(Patient shakes his head.)* Ug.

Mrs. Z. Well, let's see. *(She picks up a mirror and places it before him.)*

Patient. (Disgusted) Uh.

Mrs. Z. Ok, let's see you comb your hair. *(He does so with his left hand akwardly.)* Very good. Now imagine you are going visiting. Here is a bell. *(He pushes it; it rings.)* Now turn the knob *(he does)*. Now open the door. *(He does—each time hesitating and making a simple sound.)*

SCENE 7

Shifts to Dr. Zankel

Dr. Zankel. And thus the patient is taught to do things with his left hand, feed himself, bathe, shave, dress, undress, and all the people working with the patient on the ward are asked to cooperate and not do things for the patient, but let him do as much as possible for himself. But now the time has come that bed patients and wheelchair patients dream of when they can walk again. So let's go to Corrective Therapy, where Mr. C will show us how it's done.

SCENE 8

Parallel bars; patient in wheelchair. Mr. C near him.

Mr. C. Hello, Jack. How are you?

Patient. Uh.

Mr. C. Ready for your exercise?

Patient. Uh.

Mr. C. O.K., now let's see what you can do. Raise your left hand. *(He does so).* Now raise your right hand. *(He shows just a slight trace.)* Now raise your left leg. *(He does so.)* Now against my resistance. *(He does so.)* Now raise your right leg. *(He does so, and it goes into clonus.)* Good. Now Jack, how would you like to try to walk? *(He nods vigorously.)* OK. *(He wheels him to parallel bars and assists him in standing up.)* Now move your left hand forward and grab the bar. *(He does.)* Now your right leg. *(He does.)* Left leg. *(He does.)* Now slide your right hand on the bar, but don't try to hold it. Now, again, your left hand, your right leg. Now try your right hand, left leg, left hand, right leg, right hand, left leg. . . .

Dr. Zankel. Left hand, right leg, right hand, left leg, left hand, right leg, right hand, left leg, until finally the patient learns the rhythm and can go on, on his own. Another month goes by. The patient has been going to P.T., O.T. and C.T. and Speech. Oh, yes, I hadn't mentioned speech therapy. Well, this is a rather unique section in our hospital. For while it is located in O.T., it is run by, yes, volunteers; these fine people come to the hospital every day from 1:00 to 2:00 P.M. and help our patients to meet the outside world and to learn to communicate again. Let's go in and observe one of these sessions. The lady in charge today is Mrs. V.

SCENE 9

Speech therapy. Patient in wheelchair, "language master" between patient and Mrs. V.

Mrs. V. *(Shows patient pencil.)* What is this? *(He shakes his head.)* Say "pencil."
Patient. "e-ill."
Mrs. V. "Pen-cil."
Patient. "en-ill."
Mrs. V. Good, but I believe you can do even better. Now close your lips and say "p-p-p-p-."
Patient. "P-pp-en-il."
Mrs. V. Again, slowly, "p-p-p."
Patient. "p-p-p."
Mrs. V. "Pen."
Patient. "p-p-p-en."
Mrs. V. "s----h."
Patient. "s-ss,"
Mrs. V. "sil."
Patient. "sil."
Mrs. V. Now, "pen-cil."
Patient. "en-il."
Mrs. V. It'll come. Now, let's see what you can do with this. Here is a book, a box, and a bag. See?
Patient. Eh.
Mrs. V. Please pick up the book. *(He does.)* Put it down. *(He does.)* Now pick up the box. *(He picks up the book.)* I said the box; this is the box. *(He throws the book on the floor. She says nothing, but picks up the book and puts it down.)* Now pick up the box. *(He does.)* That's fine. *(He starts to cry. She waits patiently.)*
Dr. Zankel. This is called "thalamic crying." You notice Mrs. V pays no attention to it, and she is right. *(He stops crying.)*
Mrs. V. Shall we continue? *(She goes through a list of three cards with the "language master" until Dr. Zankel's voice breaks it up.)*
Dr. Zankel. Isn't she wonderful? We surely appreciate the fine work these and all other volunteers are doing for our patients. What would we do without them? Now you've noticed the patient is getting along pretty well; in fact, he is getting a little restless and wants to be discharged. Here he is talking to Dr. X.

SCENE 10

Back to bed scene, patient sitting in wheelchair at bedside.

Patient. Go home?
Dr. X. You want to go home. Well, you're not ready.
Patient. Home.

Dr. X. O.K. Let's see. You have a little country store, don't you? And no doubt you will want to go down and help take care of it.

Patient. Eh.

Dr. X. O.K., let's hear you count—one, two . . ."

Patient. (Counts from one to ten and hesitates once or twice.)

Dr. X. Now, let's hear you count backwards. "Ten . . ."

Patient. Ten, ten. . . .

Dr. X. I see. Now suppose I went to your store and I bought something for forty-nine cents, and I gave you a dollar. How much change would you give me?

Patient. Eh, eh *(and he gives up).*

Dr. X. I think we had better keep you here a little while longer, Besides, we want to try and do a little more for that arm.

Scene 11

Switch to Dr. Zankel.

Dr. Zankel. That arm. Most of us are inclined to give up on the arm, perhaps a little too soon. Many methods of treatment have been developed recently to help recovery in a paralyzed spastic extremity. Here Miss Y, our P.T., is showing one of them.

Scene 12

P.T., sinusoidal machine; electrodes and cords connected. Miss Y is applying the electrodes, *one to arm, one to forearm.*

Miss Y. Now remember, when you feel the current and the muscles contract, you try and help them move. Understand?

Patient. Eh.

Miss Y. O.K., now let's see you do it. *(With each contraction the patient tries. This is done two times.)*

Scene 13

Switch to Dr. Zankel.

Dr. Zankel. This is called "stimulation assistive exercise," "S.A.E.," for short. The nice part about it is that it can be given at home under a doctor's supervision. It is followed by pulley exercise and by occupational therapy. Which reminds me, you haven't as yet seen our patient receiving his O.T., so let us go back to O.T. and Mrs. Z.

Scene 14

O.T.—patient's right hand in sling.

Mrs. Z. Now, Mr. Lynn, we must keep on exercising that weak right arm. So, let's try a little sanding again. *(Patient does so, using both hands, his left hand doing most of the work.)* Enough of that. Now suppose we go back to the loom. *(She and patient go through a few steps of weaving.)*

Dr. Zankel. Thank you, Mrs. Z, and *(to public)* if you should visit O.T., you would see our patients working with leather, ceramics, wood work, metal work, arts, and other media. But now it's time to go back to corrective therapy and see how Mr. Lynn is getting along with his ambulation.

SCENE 15

C.T.—patient in wheelchair, parallel bars to one side. Mr. C. near him.

Mr. C. O.K., Jack, let's see what you can do. *(Patient gets up from wheelchair, between the parallel bars, holds on to bars, and walks without any trouble.)* Now let's try it again, with the cane. *(He gives Jack the cane, and again he walks between the parallel bars without any difficulty.)* Now, you are ready for the next step. Let's come out into the open. Would you like that?

Patient, Eh.

Mr. C. O.K., but take it easy.

Patient. Eh. *(He starts walking outside the bars, takes one perfect step, gets careless, and starts falling. Mr. C. catches him.)*

Mr. C. Let's try again, back in the parallel bars. *(He starts again.)*

SCENE 16

Back to Dr. Zankel.

Dr. Zankel. Yes, we try and try again until the patient has enough self-confidence and proper balance so that he can walk on level ground, up and down the steps, up and down an incline, so that he can meet the demands of daily living. Another month passes. All the disciplines available and indicated are utilized toward the patient's rehabilitation. Some of our patients have no home to go to, and we have to make appropriate provisions. Some have lost their jobs or have to change their jobs, and we refer them to vocational rehabilitation for training, or to the Employment Security Commission for a job. Mr. Lynn has a home and job, so he is no problem from these standpoints. And so, one morning we look in on him as he and Dr. X are discussing the problems of discharge.

SCENE 17

Dr's. Office.

Dr. X. Come in, Jack, and sit down. *(Patient walks in with cane and sits down.)* How are you getting along?

Patient. Fine.

Dr. X. How would you like to go home?

Patient. Wanted to go home month ago.

Dr. X. But you weren't ready a month ago.

Patient. Ready now.

Dr. X. All right, your heart, lungs, blood pressure are O.K., but let's see you walk. *(He does so without difficulty.)* How about holding up the cane.

(He does, and still walks O.K.) All right, sit down again. Let's hear you count.

Patient. One, two, three. . . .

Dr. X. Backwards, start with ten.

Patient. Ten, nine, eight, seven, six, five, four *(rushing)*, three, two, one.

Dr. X. If I went to your store and bought something for $1.48 and gave you $5, how much change would I get?

Patient. (thinks) $3.52.

Dr. X. O.K. I'll check with Dr. Zankel, and if he approves, you can go home on Friday. O.K.?

Patient. Fine. *(Gets up, starts walking with cane, raises cane, turns around, and walks out.)*

Scene 18

Shifts to Dr. Zankel.

Dr. Zankel. Patient did go home and has been doing well; in fact, he is here now—I mean the real Jack Lynn, whose real name is Clyde Edgerton. Would you like to say hello to the folks, Clyde?

Clyde. Hello.

Dr. Zankel. How about showing us how you walk. *(He does.)* Thanks. Jack Lynn, or Clyde Edgerton, had a place to go to and a job. But not all handicapped folks are so fortunate. Many of our handicapped people with excellent ability find the doors closed. Here is one of them. Paul Devore went through a similar program to what you have seen, and Paul can work, but he has been on the Security Commission roll for a year now, but so far no job offers. Is there anyone who will give Paul Devore a chance?— and all the other physically handicapped who are able to work? Please. Thank you.

Announcer. Thank you, Dr. Zankel. Ladies and gentlemen, you have just heard a dramatization titled, *From Bed to Job,* written and narrated by Dr. Harry T. Zankel, Chief, Physical Medicine and Rehabilitation Service, Veterans Administration Hospital, Durham, North Carolina. It was directed by Don Trotter. The dramatization was produced by Dr. Zankel in connection with Employ-the-Handicapped Week. Employ the handicapped this week and every week. It is good business. Keep in touch with your Employment Security Commission. Good night.

THE END

APPENDIX B

SOME SOURCES FOR EQUIPMENT FOR THE DISABLED

1. Be OK Self-help aids, Be OK Sales Company, Box 32, Brookfield, Illinois, 60513.
2. Cleo Living Aids, 3957 Mayfield Road, Cleveland, Ohio.
3. Fashion Able Aids (for handicapped women), Helen Gallagher, Foster House, 6523 North Galena Road, Peoria, Illinois, 61601.
4. Everest and Jennings, Inc., 1803 Pontius Avenue, Los Angeles, California, 90025.
5. General Medical Equipment Corporation, Division of Lum, Inc., Bayshore, New York.
6. Posturecheck Orthopedic Equipment Products, Sharon Hill, Pennsylvania, 19079.
7. J. A. Preston Company, 71 Fifth Avenue, New York, New York 10003.
8. Vocational Guidance and Rehabilitation Services, 2239 East 55th Street, Cleveland, Ohio, 44103.
9. For rental of equipment, consult Abbey Rents, 3112 Piedmont Road, Atlanta, Georgia, 30305.

APPENDIX C

A.D.L. (ACTIVITIES OF DAILY LIVING) PUBLICATIONS

1. American Heart Association, 44 East 23 Street, New York, New York, 10010.
   Do It Yourself Again: Self-Help Devices for the Stroke Patient.
   Strokes, A guide to the Family, EM 204.
   Up and Around, EM 358.
2. American Rehabilitation Foundation (Kenny Institute), 1800 Chicago Avenue, Minneapolis, Minnesota.
   701. *Bed Positioning Procedures.*
   702. *Transfers for Patients with Acute and Chronic Conditions.*
   703. *Range of Motion Exercise: Key to Joint Mobility.*
   704. *Self-care Homemaking for the Hemiplegic.*
   705. *Assistive Devices for the Handicapped.*
   706. *A Handbook for Rehabilitation Nursing Techniques in Hemiplegia.*
   707. *Ambulation: A Manual for Nurses.*
   709. *Language Problems after a stroke—A guide to Communication.*
   710. *Homemaking Aids for the Disabled.*
   711. *Nursing Care of the Skin.*
   713. *Wheelchair Selection: More than choosing a chair with wheels.*
   714. *Care of Patients with Bowel and Bladder Problems: A Nursing Guide.*
   719. *Braces—A Primer for Nurses.*
3. United States Government Printing Office, Washington, D.C., 20402.
   Up and Around, no. 1120 (same as American Heart Association, but larger edition).

274

APPENDIX D

ADDITIONAL BIBLIOGRAPHY ON STROKE REHABILITATION

1. Barrow, J. G.: *A Comprehensive Stroke Rehabilitation Program for Georgia* (mimeographed proposal). Atlanta, Georgia, Georgia Department of Public Health, 1959.
2. Benton: *Behavioral Change in Cerebrovascular Disease.* Harper and Row.
3. Brunnstrom, S.: *Movement Therapy in Hemiplegia.* Harper and Row.
4. *Cerebrovascular Disorders (Strokes),* PHS Pub. no. 1110. Bethesda, Maryland (20014), Information Office, National Institute of Neurological Diseases and Blindness, National Institute of Health.
5. DeForest, R. E.: *Proceedings of the National Stroke Congress, Rehabilitation, Management, Prevention.* Springfield, Thomas.
6. *Equipment for the Disabled,* 2nd Ed. Rehabilitation International, 219 East 44 Street, New York, New York, 10017, 800 pp., $20.00.
7. Fowlkes, B. H.: *Syllabus of Rehabilitation Methods and Techniques.* Highland View Hospital, Cleveland, Ohio, 44122.
8. Hirschberg, L. T.: *Rehabilitation, A Manual for the Care of the Disabled and Elderly.* Lippincott.
9. Knott, M., and Voss, D. E.: *Proprioceptive Neuromuscular Facilitation Patterns and Techniques,* 2nd Ed. Harper and Row.
10. Krusen, Kottke, and Ellwood: *A Handbook of Physical Medicine and Rehabilitation.* W. B. Saunders.
11. Licht, S.: *Rehabilitation and Medicine* (assisted by Herman J. Kamenetz). Physical Medicine Library, Elizabeth Licht, Publisher, vol. 10 (also vol. 3, *Exercise,* and vol. 9, *Orthotics*).
12. Lowman, E. W.: *Aids to Independent Living.* McGraw-Hill.
13. Miller, D. B.: *The Extended Care Facility.* McGraw-Hill.
14. *A National Program to Conquer Heart Disease, Cancer and Stroke.* Report to the President, Supt. of Documents, United States Government Printing Office, Washington, D.C., 20402.
15. Rusk, H. A.: *Rehabilitation Medicine,* 2nd Ed., C. V. Mosby and Company.
16. Millikan, Clark H. (Ed.): *Stroke, A Journal of Cerebral Circulation.* Bimonthly publication of the American Heart Association, 443 East 23 Street, New York, New York, 10010.
17. Taylor, M. L.: *Understanding Aphasia, A Guide for Family and Friends.* Institute of Physical Medicine and Rehabilitation, New York University

Medical Center, 400 East 34th Street, New York, New York 10010.

18. Ullman, M.: *Behavioral Changes in Patients following Strokes*. Charles C Thomas, 1962.

In addition to above, particularly for public reading:

19. Longerich, Mary C.: *Helping the Aphasic to Recover his Speech; A Manual for the Family*. Mary C. Longerich, Ph.D., 2007 Wilshire Boulevard, Los Angeles, California, 90057, 8 pp. fifty cents (paper).

20. Gardner, Warren H.: *Left-Handed Writing: Instruction Manual Prepared for Use in the School, Clinic or Home*. Warren H. Gardner, Cleveland Clinic Foundation. Interstate Printers and Publishers, Danville, Illinois, 61832, 29 pp., sixty cents (paper).

AUTHOR INDEX

(Note: The figures in parentheses represent numbered references)

SUBJECT INDEX